The Injured Hand

H. R. MITTELBACH

The Injured Hand

A Clinical Handbook for General Surgeons

Includes 210 illustrations

Translated by Terry Telger

Springer-Verlag
New York   Heidelberg   Berlin

H. R. Mittelbach, M.D.
Chefarzt der chirurg. Abteilung
des Städtischen Krankenhauses
6780 Pirmasens
West Germany

Library of Congress Cataloging in Publication Data

Mittelbach, Hans Reiner.
  The injured hand.

  Translation of Die verletzte Hand.
  Includes index.
  1. Hand—Wounds and injuries.   2.   Hand—
Surgery.   I.   Title.   [DNLM: 1.   Hand injuries.
WE830 M682v]
RD559.M5713   617'.575   79-219

Title of the German Original Edition: *Die verletzte Hand.* Springer-Verlag
Berlin   Heidelberg   New York, 1977.

Printed in the United States of America.

The use of general descriptive names, trade names, trademarks, etc., in this
publication, even if the former are not especially identified, is not to be taken as
a sign that such names, as understood by the Trade Marks and Merchandise
Marks Act, may accordingly be used freely by anyone.

9 8 7 6 5 4 3 2 1

ISBN 0-387-**90365**-8 Springer-Verlag New York Heidelberg Berlin
ISBN 3-540-**90365**-8 Springer-Verlag Berlin Heidelberg New York

Foreword

A specialist in hand surgery will not be available at all hospitals for some years. In the meantime, the fate of the patient will continue to rest in the hands of the surgeon who first treats him. It is essential, therefore, that both the novice and the accomplished surgeon have a sound grasp of the diagnostic and therapeutic fundamentals of hand surgery.

The material in this book is presented in a clear, practical manner by a general surgeon who has successfully practiced hand surgery; the result is an especially useful and rewarding book. Many acute situations in hand surgery are not as complicated as they appear to be, whereas other problems can be handled only after much study and experience.

Based on his experience with over 7000 general and emergency operations yearly at the Ludwigshafen Surgical Clinic and after years of intensive work in the field of hand surgery, my medical chief, Dr. H. R. Mittelbach, has taken the time and trouble to write this handbook for general and clinical practice. For the practicing surgeon and especially the resident, the most important aspects of the treatment of hand injuries have been presented in a clear, concise manner. The didactic excellence of the material, its novel format, and the simple yet forceful drawings that obviate lengthy text descriptions enable the reader to become quickly oriented.

However, the book is more than just a "cookbook" for quick reference. It also provides instructive reading for the general surgeon who wishes to become more familiar with the subject of hand surgery. Overly specialized material has been purposely omitted. Based on my own experience in the clinic and in the classroom, I believe that this book will be an excellent guide for the general surgeon.

Heinz Gelbke

Preface

Marc Iselin wrote that a shattered hand or a very serious hand injury is no longer in the province of the general surgeon, who, especially in his early years, lacks the knowledge necessary to assess the eventual consequences. One is tempted to agree with this assertion when one realizes that the young surgeon on night duty, who can generally handle problems in abdominal surgery, may be hard pressed to deal with even minor hand injuries. This is more a problem of inadequate or half-hearted training than a lack of interest, inasmuch as the treatment of hand injuries continues to be regarded as "minor surgery." Hence the call for the specialist, and rightly so. However, it is doubtful whether the specialist alone is capable of solving the problem of hand surgery, since for organizational and personal reasons most fresh hand injuries will continue to come before the general surgeon and his assistants. Even Iselin concedes that it would be better for the time being to teach the general surgeon what hand surgery is than to train hand specialists "who are motivated by an inner call and external circumstances" and who, one might add, will then wish to earn a living.

Thus, the young surgeon must learn how to examine a hand injury correctly and thoroughly. In view of the complex structure of the hand, this is no easy task. He must master many techniques for the care of each anatomical substrate and must know what treatment to administer immediately and what can be deferred. He must recognize the possibilities of subsequent reconstructive surgery, which is best left to the specialist, and must therefore preserve important structures during primary treatment. At the same time, he should recognize what structures must be sacrificed so as not to jeopardize remaining functions. He must have the courage and imagination to cope successfully with novel situations. He must understand that, where the hand is concerned, function ranks above appearance, and he must learn to recognize his own limits. It will quickly become apparent that such skills cannot be acquired without a profound knowledge of general surgery.

It is to these points that this book is addressed. It is based on my 20-year experience as a general surgeon with a career-long interest in hand surgery. It is therefore written primarily for the young surgeon who is confronted with hand injuries that he may or may not be prepared to deal with. He would do well to have this book readily available during night duty for reference. Thanks are due to the publisher for recognizing his needs.

The "specialist," on the other hand, can lay this book aside. It will teach him nothing new, and he is likely to find it incomplete. This statement is based largely on the fact that, at present, as continual progress is made in the field of hand surgery and there is a general trend toward the increased operative treatment of injuries, conservative and simple operative (and thus lower risk) forms of treatment are unjustly threatened with extinction.

This book may be regarded as a reference book that covers only those procedures and techniques that my own experience with hand surgery has shown to be practicable even by less experienced surgeons. For didactic reasons, the basic rules of hand surgery have been repeated where they apply. Bibliographic citations have been purposely held to a minimum, but they are sufficient to enable the interested reader to pursue a given subject. More exhaustive information can be obtained from the *Bibliography of Surgery of the Hand* published by the American Society for Surgery of the Hand.

The fact that this book is already in its third printing in Germany and the reports that it has enabled even younger assistants to acquire a remarkable feel for difficult procedures in the operating room have confirmed the concept behind this book.

I wish to express my thanks to my first teacher, Professor Hilgenfeldt of Bochum, the pioneer of hand surgery in the German-speaking world, who taught me the principles of hand surgery within the context of general surgery, and to Professor Gelbke of Ludwigshafen/Rhein, who gave me ample opportunity to turn these principles into reality at a large general surgical clinic where accident surgery and reconstructive surgery are still routinely practiced.

H. R. Mittelbach

Contents

Contents

Functional Anatomy and Diagnostics in Hand Surgery

In hand surgery, as in general surgery, diagnosis precedes treatment. This fact is often forgotten. The relatively simple access to the numerous densely arranged, functionally important structures tempts one to postpone the diagnosis of fresh open injuries until the operative phase of the treatment, at which time the appropriate measures are taken "according to the conditions found." Closed injuries are frequently dismissed as trivial by a glance at an unremarkable x-ray. This practice needlessly jeopardizes the function of the hand, which cannot always be restored even by costly and time-consuming reconstructive measures.

Hand surgery only *appears* to be "minor surgery," otherwise there would be no hand specialists. However, because most hand injuries are, and will continue to be, treated initially by nonspecialists—a fact which is unchanged by the "delayed operation" concept to be discussed later— every practitioner of surgery should recall the important morphological details of the hand *before* treating the hand injury and should not hesitate to refer to an anatomical atlas in order to arrive at an accurate preoperative diagnosis. Only in this way can grave errors be avoided. A thorough knowledge of hand morphology is essential. Why else does the phrase "injury of the superficial extensor tendon of the index finger" appear again and again in examination reports, and why are nerve lesions or closed ligament injuries so often overlooked?

The knowledge of hand morphology is not enough, however, for the successful practice of hand surgery. Equally important is an understanding of the interaction of the various morphological structures and the function of the human hand as an organ of grasp and touch.

I. Functional Anatomy of the Hand

The coordination of its supportive and motor functions with its sensory functions makes the hand an organ of grasp and touch. All the posi-

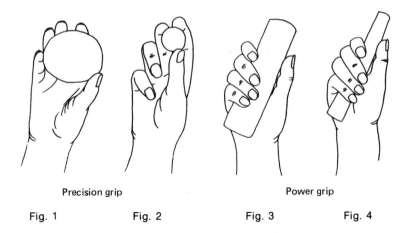

Precision grip   Power grip

Fig. 1   Fig. 2   Fig. 3   Fig. 4

tions that the hand assumes in grasping an object derive from two basic forms: the precision grip and the power grip (Napier) (Figures 1–4).

The *precision grip* grasps an object between the flexor surfaces, generally the bulbs of the fingers, with the long fingers in opposition to the thumb and a counterpressure provided by abduction. The wrist joint is stabilized in moderate expansion. The number of long fingers involved depends on the size of the object. The thumb plays an essential role in this grip.

In the *power grip* the object is held only by the partially flexed long fingers. The thumb and thenar eminence lie more or less adducted in the volar plane and control the direction in which the force is exerted. The wrist is fixed in the intermediate position with a slight inclination toward the ulnar side.

For the precision grip to be executed properly, sensation is essential for all the digits involved. In the power grip, sensation is needed at least in the thumb, which acts as the controlling element. Neither grip can be executed without participation of the thumb. We can thus appreciate the central importance of the opposable thumb in surgery of the hand.

Zur Verth has devised a more practical system for classifying grips according to four primary forms: the pinch grip, key grip, gross grip, and hook grip (Figures 5–8).

This system is useful in describing remaining functions or functions restored by reconstructive surgery and thus tells us something about the functional value of the hand.

A. Supportive and Motor Apparatus

If we consider Napier's basic forms of grasp, we see that three more or less mobile elements of the hand (namely, the thumb and first metacar-

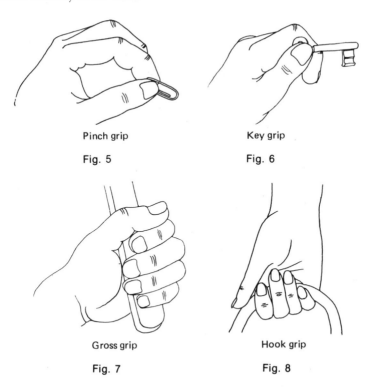

Pinch grip

Fig. 5

Key grip

Fig. 6

Gross grip

Fig. 7

Hook grip

Fig. 8

pal, the index finger, and the functionally linked third through fifth fingers with the fourth and fifth metacarpals) are grouped about a central fixed unit comprised of the distal row of carpal bones and the second and third metacarpals (Figure 9).

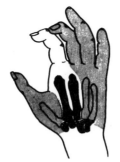

Fig. 9

1. Fixed Central Unit of the Supportive Apparatus

The skeletal members of this unit (the distal row of carpal bones and the second and third metacarpals) possess only a small range of movement due to the presence of tight ligaments. The entire unit is moved or fixed as needed by the major wrist muscles inserted into the second and third metacarpals (the radial flexor and the short radial extensor of the wrist) and thus serves as the operating base for the mobile parts of the hand.

The carpal bones form the transverse carpal arch, which is held together by the transverse carpal ligament. From this arch the longitudinal arch of the hand arises, which includes the phalanges via the second and third metacarpals.

Opposing the static transverse carpal arch is the dynamic transverse metacarpal arch, which is formed when the thenar muscles supplied by the median nerve and the hypothenar muscles supplied by the ulnar nerve contract and, owing to the loose fourth and fifth carpometacarpal joints and the transverse capitular ligaments, produce an approximation of the thumb and hypothenar.

2. Dynamic Elements of the Supportive Apparatus

a. Thumb Ray

Nine muscles, five short and four long, enable the thumb to exercise its central function during grasping:

Short Muscles of the Thumb	Long Muscles of the Thumb
First dorsal interosseous	Long extensor
Adductor	Short extensor
Short abductor	Long abductor
Short flexor	Long flexor
Opposing	

The thumb ray owes its high mobility to the saddle joint, which allows it to swivel from adduction to full opposition, the most important motors being the opposing muscle, the superficial head of the short flexor of the thumb, and the short abductor of the thumb. These muscles are supplied by the median nerve, while the remaining short muscles of the thumb are supplied by the ulnar nerve.

b. Index Finger

The index finger plays the most important interactive role with the thumb owing to the relative independence of its movements by three short and four long muscles.

c. Third through Fifth Fingers and Fourth and Fifth Metacarpals

Owing to the hypothenar muscles (short flexor of the little finger, abductor, and opposing), these elements form the true opponent of the thumb in the gross grip. The activity of the long fingers is controlled by the long extensors (common extensor of the fingers and the second and fifth extensor proprius) and flexors (superficial and deep flexors), as well as by the short interosseous and lumbrical muscles. The common extensor of the fingers and third through fifth deep flexor muscles can act only in common, because their tendons arise from muscle bellies which are continuous. The remaining muscles give the associated finger a certain degree of independent motion.

When we speak of extensors and flexors, we must realize that these seemingly clearly defined anatomical terms assume a somewhat different aspect within the context of the functional anatomy of the hand:

The wrist flexors, finger extensors, and finger abductors are synergists.
The wrist extensors, finger flexors, and finger adductors are synergists.
The interosseous and lumbrical muscles act both as finger flexors (basal joint) and finger extensors (middle and terminal joints).

3. Joints

The numerous and varied positions that the hand skeleton must assume in order to fulfill the requirements of prehension are made possible by its high degree of articulation. The radiocarpal joint, in which the first row of carpal bones articulates with the lower end of the radius, where it joins with the ulna via a fibrocartilage pad, contains an additional clearance for articular motion. The relatively loose ligamentous connections between the scaphoid, lunate, and triquetrum, which allow a certain intrinsic mobility, and the mobility of the fourth and fifth carpometacarpal joints are opposed by the rigid block created by the fixed central unit of the supportive apparatus.

Of special importance is the first carpometacarpal joint, a saddle joint which, owing to its great freedom of motion, is the "key joint" of the thumb.

The finger joints, consisting of the metacarpophalangeal (basal) joints and the proximal and distal interphalangeal (middle and terminal) joints, have essentially the same structures. The basal joint is of the condyloid type, and its range of motion is limited by the ligament apparatus. Its collateral ligaments are eccentrically arranged so that they are taut in the flexed position but slightly lax in the extended position. They tend to shorten, therefore, when they are immobilized in this position (Figure 10a–c). In addition to the ligament apparatus, these joints are also stabilized by the interosseous muscles, which can carry out this function with no assistance from the ligaments if necessary.

The middle and terminal joints are of the ginglymoid type. Due to the extremely tight capsular ligament apparatus and the insertion of the lateral ligaments at the center of rotation of the phalangeal heads, these

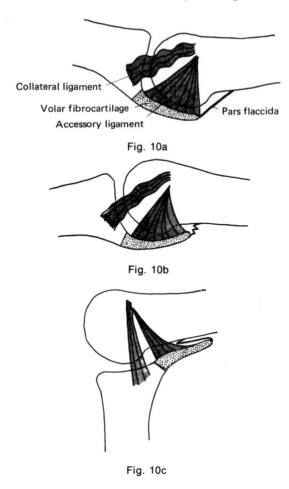

Collateral ligament

Volar fibrocartilage

Accessory ligament

Pars flaccida

Fig. 10a

Fig. 10b

Fig. 10c

joints are incapable of lateral movement in any position. The volar fibro-cartilage limits the hyperextensibility of all the joints to varying degrees.

B. Sensation

1. Superficial Sensation

Normal cutaneous sensation, or tactile gnosis, with its fine ability to discriminate among different tactile qualities, textures, shapes, and consistencies, gives the hand an important place among the sense organs. Only by virtue of its refined sensory qualities is the simple organ of grasp capable of "grasping" in the figurative sense. In terms of sensation, the thumb, index, and middle finger, supplied by the median nerve, are

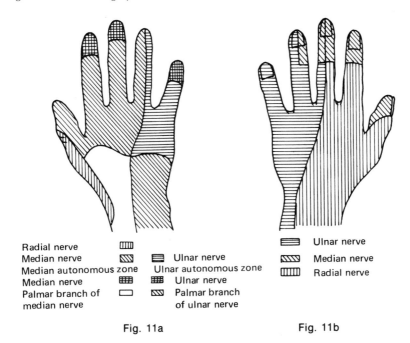

Radial nerve   ⊞
Median nerve   ▨   ⊟ Ulnar nerve
Median autonomous zone   Ulnar autonomous zone
Median nerve   ⊞   ⊞ Ulnar nerve
Palmar branch of   ▭   ▨ Palmar branch
median nerve   of ulnar nerve

⊟ Ulnar nerve
▨ Median nerve
⊞ Radial nerve

Fig. 11a   Fig. 11b

more important than the ulnar part of the hand, which is supplied by the ulnar nerve. Radial nerve sensation becomes important only if median nerve sensation is lost, at which point secondary forms of grasp are formed with the often remarkably extensive radial-sensory areas on the surface of the thumb and index finger (Figure 11a,b).

2. Deep Sensation

Equally important for hand function is deep sensation, which not only signals the position of the joints, but also plays a role in the transmission of organic sensation. Its significance in plastic operations, such as the Hilgenfeldt thumb and Littler-Zrubecky flaps, is also mentioned in passing.

II. Diagnosis in Hand Surgery

A systematic examination procedure, combined with an accurate knowledge of normal hand topography and functional anatomy, is the best prevention against an inadequate or incorrect diagnosis. It is advantageous for practically all tests to be performed by *one* examiner, with the exception of the x-ray examination and neurological consultation.

> **As a rule, an injury of the hand is not examined, but rather the hand is examined for injuries.**

Precise written documentation of test findings is a medical as well as legal necessity. It is accurate only if made during the examination procedure and supplemented by drawings of amputations, wounds, or scars as well as x-ray films. The use of a dictaphone facilitates these tasks, as does the taking of function photographs.

A. Procedure for Examining Fresh Injuries

1. General History

Metabolic diseases, circulatory disorders, previous accidents, occupation and jobs done at the workplace, and right- or left-handedness are noted.

2. Special History

Circumstances of the accident and the accident mechanism are recorded.

3. X-ray Examination of the Whole Hand
(Standard Planes)

Bone injuries, dislocations, and pathology unassociated with the accident are looked for.

4. Skin and Wound

Cuts, lacerations, crush injuries, depth of wound, skin defects, nature and extent of contamination, and circulatory conditions are noted.

5. Tendons

a. Appearance
Divisions can be detected even in the resting hand by the abnormal position of a finger relative to adjacent healthy fingers or the uninjured side.

b. Function

Simple active flexion and extension of each joint are tested. Suspected dysfunction requires further examination.

> **Wiggling movements do not demonstrate an intact tendon. Full function is the only proof!**

6. Nerves

a. Fingertip Sensation

Operative inspection of the nerves is mandatory in all injuries near the nerves. The patient's own statements are often unreliable.

b. Motor Function

Tests for motor function are indispensible in injuries of the palm, wrist, and forearm.

i. Median nerve lesion: Loss of palmar abduction of the thumb (Figure 12a,b).

ii. Ulnar nerve lesion: Loss of ability to adduct the thumb or spread the long fingers (Figure 13a,b).

7. Joint Stability

The test must be done on both hands with the proximal portion of the joint stabilized. Local anesthesia may be required.

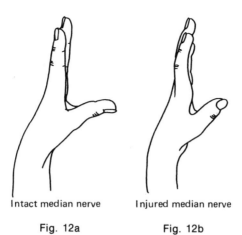

Intact median nerve   Injured median nerve

Fig. 12a   Fig. 12b

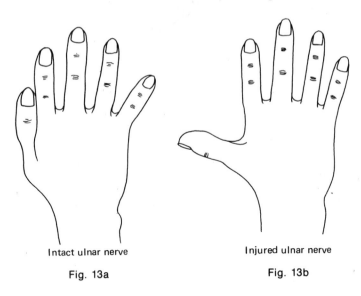

Intact ulnar nerve   Injured ulnar nerve

Fig. 13a   Fig. 13b

8. Special X-ray Examinations

Arthrograms with dental film, central carpal films, and laminagrams are obtained.

9. Tissue Vitality

A vital coloration test by dye injection (see chapter on Thermal Injuries) is performed.

B. Examination Procedure for the Preparation of Reconstructive Surgery and for Disability Evaluation

All examinations are performed on the whole arm and are compared with findings on the healthy side.

1. General History

2. Special History, Including Prior Treatments and Outcomes

3. Visual Examination

a. Scars

b. Deformities

c. Circulation

d. Swelling

e. Muscular Atrophy

f. Callosity

g. Sweat Secretion

4. Palpation

a. Test for Tenderness (Repeat with Diversion)

b. Test for Painfulness with Passive Movements

5. Motor Function

Tests of motor function provide information not only on tendon divisions, but also on neuropathy, ischemic contractures, and joint conditions. Scar contractures must be delineated. Record all data!

a. Techniques for Motor Testing

i. Active closure of fist (flexor digitorum superficialis and profundus, deep flexor tendons alone) (Figure 14)

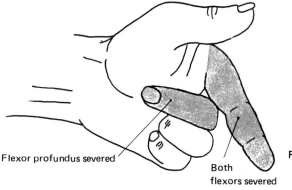

Flexor profundus severed   Fig. 14

Both
flexors severed

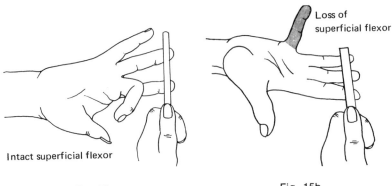

Loss of
superficial flexor

Intact superficial flexor

Fig. 15a   Fig. 15b

ii. Flexion of each finger individually, while the remaining fingers are fixed in extension to eliminate the action of the profundus tendons (superficial flexor tendon alone) (Figure 15a,b)

iii. Intrinsic muscle contracture: The middle and terminal joints can be actively flexed during flexion of the basal joint; there is no passive flexion of the middle and terminal joints when the basal joint is fixed in extension.

iv. Volkmann's contracture: There is compensation of finger flexion with increasing flexion of the wrist.

b. Typical Losses due to Tendon Divisions

i. Superficial flexor of the fingers: There is loss of flexion in the middle joint (can be tested only if profundus action is eliminated).

ii. Long flexor of the fingers: There is loss of flexion in terminal joint.

iii. Deep and superficial flexors of the fingers: There is loss of flexion in the middle and terminal joints (basal joint is flexed by interossei).

iv. Common extensor of one finger: There is slight loss of extension in the basal joint (the tendinous junctures of the adjacent fingers take over a part of the extension).

v. Common extensor of several fingers: There is loss of extension in the basal joint with free extension in the middle and terminal joints (by interossei and lumbricals).

vi. Short flexor of the thumb: There is incomplete flexion of basal joint.

vii. Long flexor of the thumb: There is loss of terminal joint flexion.

viii. Short extensor of the thumb: There is incomplete extension of the basal joint in some cases.

ix. Long extensor of the thumb: The terminal joint extension is absent or weak; the thumb ray cannot be raised above the plane of the other metacarpals.

x. Short abductor of the thumb: There is loss of palmar abduction (do not confuse with median nerve paralysis!).

xi. Long abductor of the thumb: Fingers cannot be spread in the volar plane (i.e., loss of extension in saddle joint of thumb).

c. Typical Losses due to Nerve Damage
Damage may involve disturbances of sensation and trophicity and atrophy of certain muscle groups. Be alert for trick or substitute motions!

i. Median nerve: There is loss of full rotation of the thumb ray during opposition or loss of full palmar abduction. "Oath hand" results from high median paralysis.

ii. Ulnar nerve: The long fingers cannot be spread or approximated in the volar plane when extended. There is loss of adduction of the thumb extended in the terminal joint. "Claw hand" results from high ulnar paralysis.

iii. Radial nerve: There is loss of long finger extension in the basal joints and thumb extension in the terminal joint. "Drop hand" results from high radial paralysis.

d. Techniques for Testing Sensation
These tests are very time consuming because slight discrepancies often require multiple follow-up tests. Judgments based on subjective statements by the patient, haphalgesia, or the response to hot and cold are imprecise and therefore unsuitable for surgical purposes.

i. Two-point discrimination: The points of a paper clip or caliper are applied to the fingers to determine the smallest interpoint distance at which the patient can still feel two points. The finger tested must be

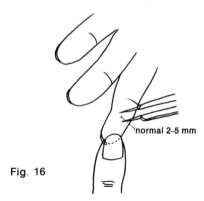

normal 2–5 mm

Fig. 16

fixed against the table top to prevent the patient from exerting counter-pressure. The test is begun with a large interpoint distance, which is gradually reduced (Figure 16).

Normal Values

Fingertip	2–5 mm
Volar surface of proximal phalanx	6–10 mm
Dorsal surface	12–15 mm

Tactile gnosis is not present if the two-point discrimination exceeds a distance of 12–15 mm. In this case only protective sensation is still present. Consistent results in 7 of 10 trials are required.

ii. Picking-up test: Small objects are picked up with and without benefit of sight. Tactile gnosis is impaired if the patient has difficulty recognizing the objects and shows poor speed and dexterity in picking them up. Watch for trick motions!

iii. Ninhydrin test (objective sensibility test of Moberg): When nerve conduction is interrupted, not only tactile gnosis is lost, but also sweat secretion due to the common course of the sympathetic and sensory nerve fibers. Thus, an affected region of the hand is dry in appearance and to the touch.

After the hands are washed to remove traces of sweat from other fingers, the bulbs of the fingers are pressed onto paper strips and the fingers are outlined in pencil. The strip is colored with a 1% solution of ninhydrin in acetone which is acidified with a few drops of acetic acid (shelf life of 2 weeks), and is then developed in an incubator for 3–5 minutes at 110°C. It can later be fixed in a 1% copper nitrate solution in

Conservative and Operative Phases of Hand Surgery

Form, sensation, and motility give the hand its physiological capabilities as we know them. It is little wonder that a fresh injury of the hand immediately raises the question of operative reconstruction. Nevertheless, the operation itself is only *one* of the pillars on which hand surgery rests. Of equal importance are the following measures:

1) The proper immobilization of the injured part.
2) The active training of all uninjured finger and arm joints.
3) The systematic, active restoration of the motility of the joints directly involved in the injury.

The scalpel, the plaster cast, and systematic therapeutic exercise (Zrubecky) are of fundamental importance for the success of hand surgery. In a broader sense, efforts to return the patient to work are an important aspect of the conservative phase of treatment. They are also part of the doctor's job.

Thus, three of the four main pillars of the treatment of hand injuries pertain to the bloodless phase. This alone demonstrates their importance, despite the fact that a disproportionate amount of attention is paid to the techniques employed during the operative phase. For this reason we shall first discuss the most important principles and techniques of the conservative phase, without which there can be no successful operative treatment.

I. Conservative Phase of Acute Hand Surgery

A. Bandaging and Immobilization

The bandage should be as small as possible but as large as necessary. The unnecessary immobilization of uninjured parts must be avoided.

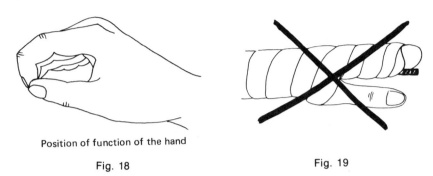

Position of function of the hand

Fig. 18   Fig. 19

With certain exceptions, the freshly injured hand is immobilized in the closed-fist position or in the "position of function," with the capsular ligaments of the joints in a stress-relieved state (Figure 18). Only in this way is muscle balance maintained and shortening of the ligaments, and thus contractures, avoided. The rare exceptions only confirm this rule. Even though this fact is generally known, violations of this basic rule are all too common, especially if bandaging is left to the nursing staff. The application of a bandage is the job of the physician.

Straight wire splints and "tongue-blade" splints have no place in the treatment of hand injuries. Constricting bandages must be avoided (Figure 19).

Circular plaster casts must be slit open (Böhler) to prevent the im-

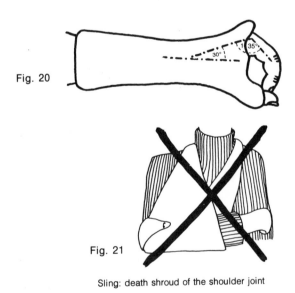

Fig. 20

Fig. 21

Sling: death shroud of the shoulder joint

pairment of blood flow. Plaster casts that do not serve to immobilize the fingers must extend at least beyond the metacarpophalangeal joints on the dorsal side so that no edema will occur on the dorsum of the hand. On the volar side they must reach no farther than the distal volar flexion crease so that the basal joints of the long fingers can be flexed (Figure 20). Casts and splints that serve to immobilize the long fingers are best applied on the dorsal side in order to avoid the inadvertent immobilization of the joints in undesired extension.

Slings should not be used. They are rightly called the "death shroud" of the shoulder joint (Figure 21). These principles also apply to the postoperative phase following reconstructive surgery.

B. Active Therapeutic Exercise

Active exercise is a good means of preventing dystrophy, joint stiffness, and contractures in many cases. All nonimmobilized finger and arm joints must be actively moved through their full range of motion from the first day on. The patient should be encouraged to perform his exercises hourly. This exercise should not be painful, and analgesic medication is desirable for the first few days. The exercise should be supervised so that the patient can be urged to overcome the initial painful resistance. Massage or the local application of heat in any form has no place in the conservative treatment of fresh hand injuries (Figure 22).

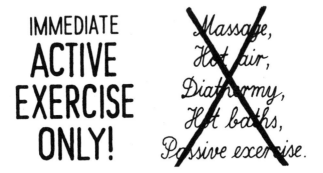

Fig. 22

II. Conservative Phase of Reconstructive Hand Surgery

Psychological as well as surgical aspects must be considered during this phase. Reconstructive surgery is impossible not only if the joints are stiff or the blood supply to the hands is impaired, but also if the patient lacks the will for rehabilitation or if a lack of intelligence or insight renders the exercise program useless. Innervation defects, a conservative domain, must be promptly distinguished from true joint stiffness. Proper psychological guidance of the patient through the reconstructive process is therefore essential. It must be begun during primary treatment, or it is usually too late. Reconstructive operations on severely damaged hands should therefore be limited to those patients who elect to undergo such surgery.

A. Active Exercise

A supervised program of active therapeutic exercise of all joints of the injured member improves not only the function of the joints but also the blood supply to injured parts. Passive exercises, on the other hand, are often painful and lead only to swelling, a reduction of blood flow, and thus impaired mobility. They are also harmful during the conservative phase of reconstructive surgery.

B. Therapeutic Splints

If the patient's own muscular strength is insufficient to effect the stretching of shortened capsular ligaments, this must be done with the aid of therapeutic splints, rather than the force of a third party. Masseurs belong to the surgery of the past. Today they have given way to

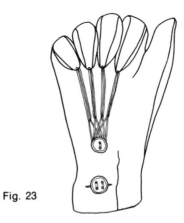

Fig. 23

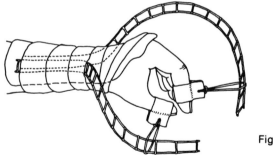

Fig. 24

physiotherapists and occupational therapists. The traction exerted by a therapeutic splint must cause no pain and must be slight enough such that active movements can be made to their full extent against the pull of the splint.

Standard therapeutic splints are available commercially. On occasion they must be custom made to suit individual needs. Unfortunately, by the time they are delivered the need for them may no longer exist, but custom-made therapeutic splints are generally unnecessary for routine practice. If we limit our concern to the recovery of standard functions, the following simple measures are adequate:

1) The long fingers can be flexed with the aid of a flexion glove. This glove is based on an idea by Krukenberg but is better known today as the Moberg glove. It can be made by the patient himself from a leather glove, buttons, and rubber bands (Figure 23).

2) Extension of the long fingers and abduction of the thumb can be attained by means of a cast with a plastered-in wire splint. The tension exerted by small elastic bands is transmitted to the fingers through felt loops. By adjusting the position of the loops, traction and countertraction can be applied at each finger joint (Figure 24).

3) The fingers can be spread by means of a rubber tube provided with an oval window, which is folded and pressed into the space at the base of two adjacent long fingers (Figure 25a,b).

C. Electrotherapy

Prior to reconstructive surgery, motor nerve injuries require appropriate electrotherapy in order to keep the reacting organs functional. After surgery they are a supportive factor in the process of instructing the patient in the use of the repaired extremity.

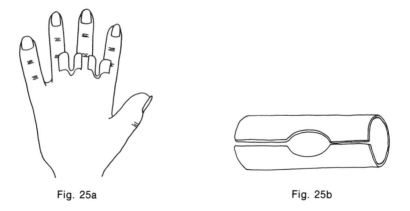

Fig. 25a   Fig. 25b

III. Vocational Rehabilitation

Severe hand injuries often leave functional disabilities that would appear to make it impossible for the patient to resume his former activities. The physician must anticipate this so that efforts at surgical and vocational rehabilitation will be made while the patient is still in the "cooperative phase." Once he has become a "hard-core pensioner" all such efforts are too late.

Surgical rehabilitation can return the patient on a full or limited basis to his former livelihood even if the injury is extremely severe. This can be done conservatively by training, or operatively by the creation of a hand remnant with some elements of grasp. Instruction by an occupational therapist is helpful in such cases.

Unfortunately, vocational rehabilitation is all too often overshadowed by the concept of "resettlement." For the younger patient, the change to a new vocation after a severe injury may be advantageous and easily mastered, but for the patient who is over 40 years old, such a change is often difficult if not impossible. We shall not explore the reasons for this here; they are numerous and lie beyond the scope of surgery. Nevertheless, experience has shown that a simple change of duties at the workplace leads in many cases to a much more satisfactory solution for all the parties involved (patient, doctor, and insurer) than does resettlement. All such measures must be instituted early on, not just at the conclusion of treatment. The surgeon is well advised to learn something about the conditions at the patient's place of employment and then confer with both patient and employer to find the best approach to vocational rehabilitation.

Bibliography

Moberg, E.: Dressings, splints and postoperative care in hand surgery. Surg. Clin. North
   Am. 44, 941 (1964).
Pap, K.: Behandlung der Fingerkontrakturen durch Diafixation. Zentralbl. Chir. 89, 51υ
   (1964).
Zrubecky, G.: Die konservative Phase in der Handchirurgie einschließlich Bandverletzun-
   gen. Z. Orthop. 99, 238 (1964).

Surgery of the Hand

The results of hand surgery have been greatly improved by the application of Bunnell's "atraumatic technique." Oversize instruments and traumatizing procedures lead to excessive cicatrization, which can severely impair normal hand function. In addition to adequate anesthesia, the following are indispensible for atraumatic hand surgery:

A bloodless operating field.
Fine instruments.
Adequate access.

I. Bloodless Field

A blood-drenched operating field makes it impossible to identify the fine, functionally important anatomical structures in the hand. The result is overlooked injuries or the iatrogenic destruction of intact structures. Continual swabbing traumatizes sensitive tissues, especially the gliding surfaces of the tendons, and leads to undesired cicatrization. Even gross contamination may go undetected.

Thus, a bloodless operating field is essential, not only for extensive fresh wounds or in major reconstructive operations, but also for minor injuries.

> All operations on the hand require either an Esmarch bandage in combination with a pneumatic cuff tourniquet or tourniquet ischemia.

A. Expression of Blood with an Esmarch Bandage

The blood is expressed by winding an Esmarch bandage from the fingertips upward under moderate tension. A blood pressure cuff is applied over the end of the Esmarch bandage and inflated to a pressure of 300 mm Hg. Commercially available devices for monitoring and maintaining the pressure facilitate this procedure. The use of an Esmarch bandage or even a rubber tube to occlude the vessels may result in injury to the brachial nerves, however, so these procedures are not recommended (Figure 26a–c). Nerve paralysis resulting from ischemia induced by other than pneumatic means constitutes malpractice according to the present law in some countries.

B. Tourniquet Ischemia

The arm is extended vertically for 2–3 minutes, the brachial artery is manually compressed, and the blood pressure cuff, which was loosely applied beforehand, is rapidly inflated to a pressure of 300 mm Hg.

C. Esmarch Bandage or Pneumatic Tourniquet?

An Esmarch bandage is basically contraindicated in the presence of infectious processes because there is a risk of bacterial contamination. The tourniquet produces a similarly bloodless field, with the added advantage that the larger vessels that are unavoidably severed during the course of the operation can be more easily detected by residual filling and can thus be promptly attended to. If performed properly, therefore, tourniquet ischemia is the procedure of choice. Both procedures can be maintained for up to 90 minutes, even for older patients. If the

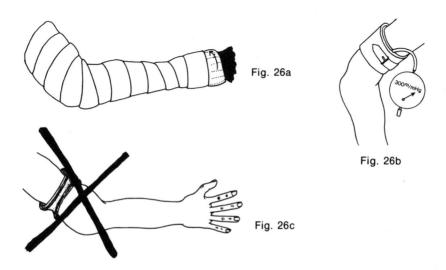

Fig. 26a

Fig. 26b

Fig. 26c

operation lasts longer, the blood flow must be restored for a few minutes and the tourniquet reapplied.

D. Finger Tourniquet

This is the *only case* in which a rubber tube can be used. The arm is held vertically for several minutes. Then a thin rubber tube is carefully wrapped around the base of the finger and fastened on the dorsal side with a large clamp (Figure 27).

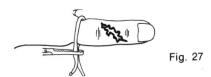

Fig. 27

The finger tourniquet is not without its dangers. If it is too tight, left on longer than 15 minutes, or used on older patients with pre-existing circulatory disorders, gangrene may result.

After the tourniquet is removed, reactive hyperemia leads to a more or less profuse bleeding. Do not employ instrumental measures to arrest the bleeding. The bleeding will stop in a few minutes if the arm is raised and mild compression is applied, if stasis due to a too tight blood pressure cuff or pressure from the drapes is avoided. Only the larger vessels then need to be ligated with 6/0 catgut or occluded by clamping or microcoagulation.

II. Instruments

The retractors, forceps, and hemostats ordinarily used in surgery are too bulky for hand surgery. They crush the tissue and thus lead to undesired scar formation. A large assortment of special instruments for hand surgery are available. While they facilitate the procedures, they are not all absolutely necessary. The only instruments that are essential are fine forceps, fine clamps, fine scissors, fine nerve hooks, and a very fine sharp scalpel. Also needed are instruments for bone surgery, including at least a drill, saw, Luer forceps, fine raspatories, Kirschner wires 0.8–1.4 mm in diameter, side cutters, and nontoothed forceps. Finally, fine (4/0–6/0) atraumatic, nonswelling suture material (steel wire or synthetic fiber) and needle forceps corresponding to the needle size are required. For

tendon repair, ready to use Lengemann sutures as well as doubly atraumatically armed sutures are available.

**For the routine operation in an emergency room it should be remembered
that any wound can be treated with fine instruments, but damage can be
inflicted on the hand with ordinary instruments.**

III. Adequate Access

The high density of the anatomical structures essential for hand and
finger function requires an operative exposure adequate to ensure that
no injuries are overlooked and that different anatomical structures are
not confused. Many avenues of approach to hand structures have
proved to be practical. They afford an optimal view of the operating
area, help prevent secondary injuries, and, if care is taken with respect to
joint creases and skin cleavage lines, prevent the scar contractures that
usually occur when the incision crosses joint creases and skin lines at
right angles and is placed under tensile and tangential stress by movements.

The following incisions are permissible:

1) All incisions that follow the cleavage lines and the joint creases or
   cross them at angles less than 60°.
2) On the finger, dorsolateral longitudinal incisions that are oriented
   along the dorsal ends of the joint flexion creases (Figure 28).

The following incisions are prohibited:

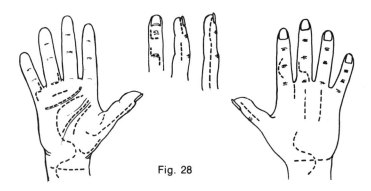

Fig. 28

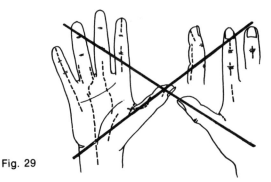

Fig. 29

1) All incisions that cross joint creases and cleavage lines at right angles.
2) All incisions that pass through the interdigital creases (Figure 29).

Extensions of wounds that must be made during treatment of a fresh injury must also follow these principles.

IV. Atraumatic Tissue Handling

Whether the hand is fixed in a "lead hand" or a similar device during the operation is left to the discretion of the surgeon. It is best in any case for an assistant to be present who can place the operating field in the position required, with the arm extended laterally on an arm board. Compressive injuries to the radial nerve must be avoided. The arm board must therefore be no higher than the plane of the operating table.

The operator can best maintain a "steady hand" during the often lengthy operations if he and his assistants are seated while working.

Any unnecessary contact with the wound surfaces must be avoided. For this reason all sutures are knotted by instrument. Holding sutures are better than hooks for maintaining operative exposure. Even Lexer is quoted as saying that he "prefers to be alone in the wound."

A bloodless operating field makes swabbing largely unnecessary. If swabbing cannot be avoided, it should be done only with moist swabs (Ringer's solution or physiological saline) to minimize tissue trauma. Harmful drying of the operating field must be prevented by occasional irrigation with Ringer's solution. This also mechanically cleans the operative wound of bacteria.

Vascular ligatures lead to undesired foreign body granulations. At the same time, postoperative hematomas must be prevented in the interest of normal healing. Hemostasis by torsion of the vessel with a fine vascular clamp is theoretically the best procedure but is not always adequate in practice. Therefore, ligature of the vessels with catgut 6/0 cannot always be avoided if the physician does not wish to resort to microcoagulation of the vascular lumen by means of an electric current.

Bibliography

Bruner, J. M.: The zig-zag volar-digital incision for flexor tendon surgery. Plast. Reconstr. Surg. 40, 571 (1967).
Verdan, C.: Basic principles in surgery of the hand. Surg. Clin. North Am. 47, 355 (1967).

Anesthesia in Hand Surgery

The production of full insensibility and perhaps even the suspension of voluntary motor function for the duration of the operation are the main prerequisites for successful hand surgery. The choice of the form of anesthesia employed depends largely on the age and condition of the patient, on the local, personal, and technical facilities available, and, equally important, on organizational constraints. Finally, it is determined by the location of the operating area and the necessity of a bloodless field.

Organizational factors, as well as the long duration of many hand operations, can limit the indication for general anesthesia. This disadvantage is offset by the fact that the upper extremities of man are remarkably amenable to selective or complete block anesthesia. This is the anesthesia of choice for the majority of ambulatory hand patients because it can be used at any time on practically any patient and leads to few immediate or delayed complications. (Remember that the patient is incapable of driving a vehicle even under the effect of a local anesthetic.)

Administration by injection about the wound is unsuitable if the evidence, location (palm, wrist), and accident analysis suggest the possibility of injuries to important deep-lying anatomical structures because this form of anesthesia permits neither an adequate wound inspection nor proper care. It can also lead to circulatory disorders, and thus the danger of infection, through the swelling of tissues. In the case of fractures, the same applies to injection of the anesthetic into the fracture hematoma.

The local anesthetic chosen should meet the following requirements:

Low toxicity.
Good tissue tolerance.
Rapid onset of action.
Long duration of action.

Anesthetics that satisfy these requirements include mepivacaine, lido-caine, and, for lengthy operations, bupivacaine.

Complications with generalized reactions may result from an intoler-ance to the anesthetic, inadvertant intravascular injection, a disregard of contraindications to epinephrine-containing solutions, or overdose.

Absolute contraindications to epinephrine-containing solutions are as follows:

1) Intravenous injection.
2) Glaucoma.
3) Paroxysmal tachycardia.
4) High-frequency absolute arrhythmia.

Relative contraindications to epinephrine-containing solutions are as follows:

1) Advanced age.
2) Arteriosclerosis.
3) Hypertension.
4) Diabetes mellitus.
5) Occlusive arterial disease (dead finger, intermittent claudication).

The dose limits for local anesthetics with and without vasoconstrictors, using lidocaine, mepivacaine, and bupivacaine as examples, are shown in Table 1.

If epinephrine-containing solutions or excessive amounts of anes-thetic are injected during Oberst's anesthesia or metacarpal block anes-thesia, local gangrene may result. Nerve irritation phenomena with hypo- and paresthesia can always occur after block anesthesia. They are

TABLE 1. Dose Limits for Local Anesthetics

Anesthetic	Concentration (%)	Without vasoconstrictor (ml)	With vasoconstrictor (ml)
Lidocaine	2	10	25
	1	20	50
	0.5	40	100
Mepivacaine	2	15	25
	1	30	50
	0.5	60	100
Bupivacaine	0.5	30[a]	
	0.25	60[a]	

[a] With and without vasoconstrictor.

more common in central forms of anesthesia and are always of a more transient nature. They are usually brought on by the piercing of a nerve and can be largely avoided by the use of fine cannulae.

> **The dose and concentration of a local anesthetic should always be as low as possible. Anesthetic can be saved by patiently waiting until the drug takes effect.**

I. Technique of Block Anesthesia

A. Oberst's Block Anesthesia at the Base of the Finger

The needle is inserted bilaterally into the base of the proximal phalanx on the dorsal side. One milliliter of the 2% solution (without epinephrine) is injected about the dorsal and volar digital nerves from a single insertion point on each side (Figure 30a,b). The onset of action takes 2–4 minutes. Aseptic surgery can then be performed on the middle joint and the two distal phalanges.

Oberst's anesthesia and tourniquet ischemia fulfill their purpose only if they are employed "reasonably and sensibly." An overdose of anesthetic can lead to gangrene of the finger just as easily as a tourniquet that is applied too tightly or left on longer than 15 minutes.

B. Metacarpal Block Anesthesia

The injections are made on the dorsum of the hand on both sides of the metacarpal bone just below its head. The dorsal and volar nerves are

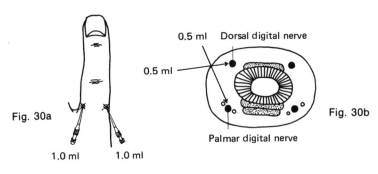

Fig. 30a   Fig. 30b

0.5 ml   Dorsal digital nerve

0.5 ml

Palmar digital nerve

1.0 ml   1.0 ml

Without vasoconstrictor

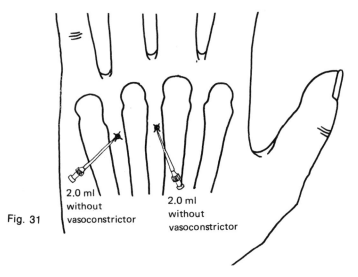

Fig. 31

2.0 ml without vasoconstrictor

2.0 ml without vasoconstrictor

blocked with 2 ml of the 2% epinephrine-free solution on each side (Figure 31), the volar nerve being reached by penetration through the interosseal space. The onset of action takes about 5 minutes. This anesthesia is suited for surgery of and distal to the basal joint. In the case of multiple finger injuries, a central form of anesthesia is recommended.

C. Block Anesthesia at the Wrist

The entire hand can be effectively anesthetized by selectively blocking the median or ulnar nerve, or both together, and the dorsoradial sensory branches of the radial nerve (Figure 11a,b). This form of anesthesia is particularly suited for concurrent surgery on several fingers if the application of a tourniquet to the basal joints is still possible. Operations in the region of the metacarpus require central anesthesia because a tourniquet is necessary.

1. Median Nerve Block

The guide for the median nerve is the tendon of the long palmar muscle. The needle is inserted radial to the palmar tendon and central to the wrist flexion creases; a subcutaneous depot is applied to block the sensory palmar branch of the median nerve; correct needle placement to block the nerve is demonstrated by sensory paresthesia in the first three fingers as the needle is inserted more deeply. Three milliliters of the 1% epinephrine-containing solution is necessary to produce anesthesia

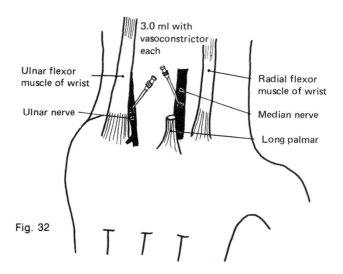

Ulnar flexor
muscle of wrist

3.0 ml with
vasoconstrictor
each

Radial flexor
muscle of wrist

Ulnar nerve

Median nerve

Long palmar

Fig. 32

(Figure 32). Blockage of the radial branches requires an additional 3 ml. Onset of action takes 5–6 minutes (Figure 33).

2. Ulnar Nerve Block

The guide here is the tendon of the ulnar flexor muscle of the wrist. The needle is inserted radial to this tendon at the level of the ulnar head until paresthesia is evoked in the little finger. The dorsal branch of the ulnar nerve is reached from the same insertion point by guiding the cannula past the ulnar head toward the dorsal side. Three milliliters of the 1% epinephrine-containing solution is required to anesthetize both branches. Onset of action takes 5–6 minutes (Figures 32, 33).

Selective anesthesia of the ulnar nerve can also be achieved by administering 3 ml of the 1% solution with epinephrine 2 cm proximal to the ulnar groove behind the ulnar epicondyle at the elbow joint. The onset of action takes about 10 minutes (Figure 34).

D. Subaxillary Block Anesthesia

As they leave the axilla at about the level of the deltoid insertion, the three large brachial nerves still occupy the same muscle groove. The guide is the brachial artery, which is easily palpable at this level. The patient is in supination, his arm raised 90° at the shoulder joint and bent 90° at the elbow joint. The brachial pulse is felt, and a slight pressure of the finger is used to gently fix the neurovascular bundle against the hu-

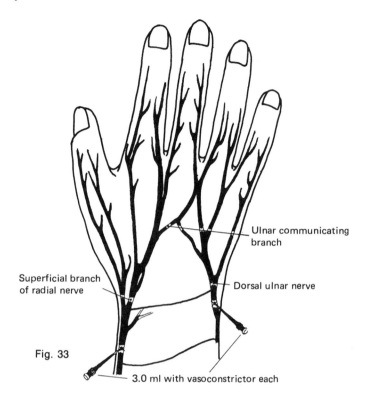

Ulnar communicating branch

Superficial branch of radial nerve

Dorsal ulnar nerve

Fig. 33

3.0 ml with vasoconstrictor each

merus. The needle is inserted over the artery (Figure 35a). Ten milliliters of the 1% anesthetic solution with epinephrine is injected ventral and dorsal to the artery in the neurovascular bundle after the surgeon is certain of the extravascular placement of the cannula (Figure 35b). The prior occurrence of paresthesia convinces the surgeon of the correct placement of the needle within the connective tissue sheath investing the nerves and vessels. The drug takes effect within 30–45 minutes. This form of block anesthesia permits surgery on the hand and forearm for up to 2.5 hours with the complete suspension of voluntary motor activity. Reinjection to prolong the anesthesia is possible, but the use of bupivacaine as a depot anesthetic is preferred.

An additional field block of the cutaneous nerves at the site of the pneumatic duff with 15 ml of a 0.5% epinephrine-containing solution is recommended. Supplementary nerve blocks in the forearm may be necessary on occasion. However, this disadvantage is fully offset by the fact that even the less experienced surgeon is unlikely to encounter complications in this type of block anesthesia. If a lengthy operation is anticipated, premedication is advised.

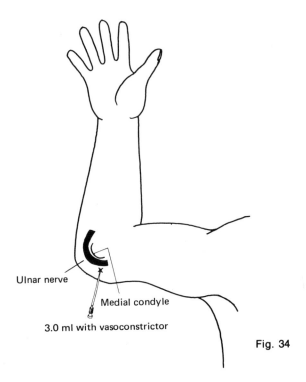

Ulnar nerve

Medial condyle

3.0 ml with vasoconstrictor

Fig. 34

E. Supraclavicular Plexus Anesthesia

Due to the danger of pneumothorax (see below) as well as other general reactions (apnea), this form of anesthesia should be employed only by the experienced operator under clinical conditions and must never be employed bilaterally. Anesthesia of the brachial plexus is done at the

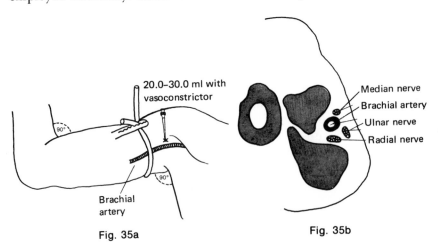

20.0–30.0 ml with
vasoconstrictor

Median nerve
Brachial artery
Ulnar nerve
Radial nerve

Brachial
artery

Fig. 35a

Fig. 35b

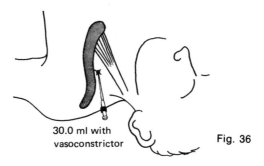

30.0 ml with
vasoconstrictor   Fig. 36

point where it passes over the first rib. The patient is in supination with his head turned toward the contralateral side. The needle, which is about 5 cm long, is inserted from the cranial side at an 80° angle 1 cm above and slightly lateral to the middle of the clavicle until contact is made with a plexus fascicle or the first rib. By "hunting" with the needle along the rib, the operator attempts to make contact with all three fascicles. Then 10 ml of anesthetic with vasoconstrictor is injected at each main trunk. The onset of action takes 30–45 minutes (Figure 36).

The following dangers may be encountered with this form of anesthesia:

1)   Pleural puncture, pneumothorax: The patient coughs or complains of shortness of breath. The anesthesia must be immediately discontinued, and stationary observation and treatment are indicated.

2)   Intravascular injection: To prevent this, careful aspiration is required before injection. If the subclavian artery is punctured, the needle has been inserted too far medially, and the plexus must be sought farther laterally (Figure 36).

F. Intravenous Block Anesthesia

This form of anesthesia, which acts by diffusion through the capillary network, is used only if ischemia can be induced in a precise, controlled manner. A double cuff with automatic pressure control is applied to the upper arm. An indwelling cannula is inserted into a well-congested forearm vein and secured there. The arm is then wrapped from the fingertips to the cuff with an Esmarch bandage. Next the proximal cuff is inflated to the 250–300 mm Hg necessary to maintain ischemia. The Esmarch bandage is removed, and 40 ml of a 0.5% solution of prilocaine without vasoconstrictor (2–3 mg/kg body weight) is rapidly injected. Careful massage of the skin accelerates the onset of action. As soon as the patient complains of pain at the proximal cuff, the distal cuff is inflated and the proximal cuff loosened. To prevent the too rapid entry of the local anesthetic into the circulation, the ischemia is continued inter-mittently by de- and inflating the cuff three to five times after the opera-tion, but no sooner than 30 minutes after injection.

This form of anesthesia is suitable for adults only (beware of known intolerance to local anesthetics) and only for operations 30–90 minutes in duration.

G. Other Anesthesias

Quite adequate for practical purposes are subaxillary block anesthesia, block anesthesia at the wrist, and metacarpal block anesthesia. Even the beginner can learn them quickly if he is familiar with the location of the nerves. He can thus create a painless operative field with no fear of com-plications.

In older patients and patients with a history of occlusive arterial dis-ease ("dead finger" and intermittent claudication), Oberst's anesthesia is contraindicated, and block anesthesia at the wrist and metacarpus must be performed with an epinephrine-free anesthetic.

In the case of children, it is in the interest of both doctor and patient that all procedures beyond the closure of a simple wound be done under general anesthesia, with strict adherence to a 6-hour interval since the last meal.

II. Treatment of Toxic Reactions to Local Anesthesia

Toxic reactions are rare if proper precautions are taken, especially with regard to dose limits and extravascular injection. Their occurrence calls for prompt action.

A. Shock

Shock is treated by the administration of oxygen, artificial respiration (intubation), lowering of the head, intravenous sympathicomimetics (e.g., norepinephrine), plasma expanders (e.g., low molecular weight dextran), and heart massage if cardiac arrest is suspected.

The puncture of a peripheral vein may be difficult or impossible dur-ing shock. The subclavian vein is always accessible. The needle is in-serted below the middle of the clavicle, with the needle tip guided in the direction of the jugular notch of the sternum (Figure 37).

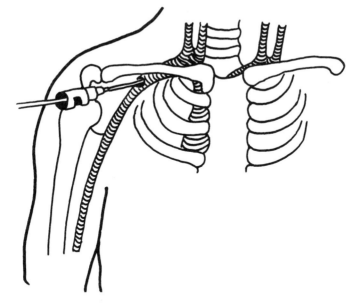

Fig. 37

B. Respiratory Insufficiency

The administration of oxygen and artificial respiration (intubation) are used to treat this reaction.

C. Convulsions

Intravenous barbiturate anesthesia and muscle relaxants are used if needed. The administration of oxygen and artificial respiration may also be necessary.

III. Treatment of Allergic Reactions to Local Anesthesia

Allergic reactions are also rare. Before the local anesthetic is administered, the patient is asked whether he has ever been given a local anesthetic and whether he reacted adversely to it. If an allergic tendency is present, general anesthesia is advised. An allergic reaction requires the administration of corticosteroids and the maintenance of vital functions (respiration, cardiac activity, and circulation).

Bibliography

Brodfield, W. J. D.: Digital block anesthesia and its complications. Brit. J. Surg. 50, 495 (1965).

Moore, D. C., Bridenbougen, L. D., Eater, K. F.: Block of the upper extremity. Arch. Surg. 90, 68 (1965).

Solonen, K. A., Tarkkonen, L.: Intravenous anesthesia in surgery of the hand. Arch. Orthop. Unfallchir. 60, 115 (1966).

Care of Open Hand Injuries

Primary healing of the wound is the basis and prerequisite for all successful hand surgery. It is the task of the surgeon to bring about primary healing by following correct procedures before, during, and after the operation.

I. Correct Procedure before the Operation

1) Contamination of the wound by resistant hospital germs is prevented by the immediate application of a sterile dressing, together with antiseptics from the hexachlorophene or quaternary ammonium-base series if need be. The hand must be wrapped in this way prior to x-ray examination. Alcohol-containing disinfectants do more harm than good through protein precipitation.

2) All finger rings must be immediately removed, whether the finger is injured or not. This is more difficult once edema has developed.

3) The application of a tourniquet is generally unnecessary even in the case of severe bleeding and usually only leads to hyperemia. Applied long before the operation, a tourniquet causes the patient unnecessary pain and shortens the tolerance time of the ischemia. In such a situation the application of a compression bandage and elevation of the injured extremity are sufficient to prevent excessive blood loss.

4) A thorough examination of the injured hand and the wound is performed with all the usual precautions observed in an aseptic operating room, including sterile clothing, gloves, masks, and head coverings.

5) Thorough cleaning of the wound as well as the arm up to the bend of the elbow is done with at least soap and water, but preferably with hexachlorophenes or quaternary ammonium bases. It must be remembered that hexachlorophenes are absorbed through the skin. The

agent must therefore be washed off, especially in the case of small children, to avoid intoxication.

6)   The sterile drapes for the operation must be applied so as to leave the entire hand and forearm exposed to ensure adequate visibility and freedom of movement. Measures must be taken to keep the drapes from shifting from the nonsterile to the sterile area.

7)   The operation must be carefully planned to eliminate time pressure during the procedure.

8)   Remember tetanus prophylaxis!

II. Immediate Care, "Delayed Primary Care," or "Emergency with Delayed Operation"?

Basically, the hand wound should be treated according to the principles of Friedrich. However, the density of functionally important anatomical structures in the hand often makes a radical Friedrich-type wound excision impossible. Nevertheless, experience has shown that with the generally good conditions of blood flow in the hand, radical wound excision can be abandoned in favor of adequate debridement, and the "8-hour limit" until the wound is cared for can be exceeded, especially in the case of severe injuries, for organizational reasons.

> **This release from the basic rules governing the operative treatment of wounds should in no way be interpreted as a license for careless work!**

With care taken to avoid iatrogenic injuries, the following procedures are performed:

1)   Devitalized skin and muscle tissue must be removed without regard for subsequent closure of the wound.
2)   Contaminated skeletal members must be cleaned with a chisel or curet.
3)   Contaminated cartilage must be cleaned.
4)   If necessary, defibrillated and contaminated portions of joint capsules and ligaments are resected for up to one-half their thickness, and dirt particles are painstakingly removed.

> **Dirty nerves, vessels, and tendons should not be removed!**

Instrumental debridement is greatly aided by the mechanical action of frequent irrigation with physiological saline or Ringer's solution.

If the operative care of a hand injury is postponed, a sharp distinction must be made between the "delayed primary care" (Scharizer) for organizational reasons and the "emergency with delayed operation" (Iselin's *urgence avec opération différée*), whose application may be determined by pathophysiologic as well as organizational factors. Both strive for a global restoration of all structures within the framework of primary operative care, as opposed to the method of Moberg, who advocates immediate, complete wound closure and the deferment of reconstructive measures.

In the delayed emergency, which in no way represents a passive waiting, the operation is postponed until at least 48 hours after the injury, by which time the swelling has subsided, the body's local defenses against infection have been mobilized, and the viability of the tissue can be clinically assessed with some degree of certainty. During this time, local antiseptic measures are taken on the elevated, immobilized extremity, and large doses of a broad-spectrum antibiotic are administered. Scharizer pursues a middle course by employing the local and general measures of Iselin, but deferring the global operation until the nearest point in time which is favorable from an organizational standpoint, and placing less emphasis on the biological aspects of edema therapy and defense reactions.

In specific cases the procedure will be determined by the surgical experience of the attending physician. Nevertheless, the following general recommendations can be offered:

1) Immediate care: all soft tissue injuries which permit primary wound closure without plastic measures.
2) Delayed primary care: all hand injuries which require an experienced surgeon who is available within 12 hours after the injury.
3) Emergency with delayed operation: only the most severe hand injuries which, for general medical reasons, require that the operation be postponed and be treated by an experienced surgeon or a specialist.

The operation can, of course, be interrupted at any time for consultation with a more experienced surgeon or referral to a specialist if the first attending physician finds that he has reached the limits of his abilities. This demands insight and self-criticism.

III. Severe Combined Injuries: Global Primary Care or Staged Reconstruction?

This question has no single answer. The type of trauma, the extent of the injury, the condition of the patient, and the attitude and experience of the surgeon are the main factors determining the choice of procedure. We usually choose staged reconstruction:

First session: skin, bones, and extensor tendons.
Second session: flexor tendons and nerves.

IV. Correct Procedure during the Operation

A. General

1) Maximum asepsis must be maintained.
2) A tissue-sparing (atraumatic) technique is used.
3) Primary wound closure is performed, employing primary plastic measures if necessary.
4) The suture must be tension free in all cases and on all substrates.
5) The extent of the injuries and the measures taken should be documented in detail during the course of the operation. Subsequent reconstructive operations can be correctly planned only if complete data are available on the damaged structures. Experience has shown that much is forgotten if the operative report is written after the operation.
6) The sutures should not be drawn too tight during closure of the wound. Even the tissue beneath the suture is viable (i.e., must receive a blood supply), even if wound edema develops (see item 4).

B. Wound Excision: Scalpel or Scissors?

The scalpel offers the advantage of a smooth-edged incision, whereas scissors are liable to crush still healthy tissue. In practice, the possibilities for the use of the scalpel are limited by the fact that more tissue most often be sacrificed than is absolutely necessary. The scissors, on the other hand, provide a surer cut if they are sharp and tightly hinged. We have found no disadvantages in the use of scissors. The decisive factor is the careful and thorough removal of contaminants and all devitalized tissue.

C. Wound Excision: When Is It Unnecessary, When Is It Necessary, and What Are the Limits?

Practice has shown that smooth and clean incised wounds that do not extend beyond the cutis generally heal by first intention without excision or even suturing if the wound is disinfected and a plaster bandage is applied. A Friedrich-type excision in such cases would enlarge the wound and increase the risk of healing by granulation.

Lacerations and crush (including superficial) wounds result in local tissue destruction and therefore require excision just as any wound extending to the subcutaneous fatty tissue. In theory, this includes gunshot and stab wounds, at which point we have already reached the practical limits of wound excision. Radical wound excision is forbidden in cases in which functionally critical structures that have retained their continuity (e.g., nerves, digital arteries, or tendons) would have to be sacrificed during the course of the operation. In such cases the surgeon must limit himself to excision of the cutaneous wound and debridement and irrigation of the rest of the wound.

D. Primary Suture versus Delayed Primary Suture

1. Primary Suture

As a rule, a cleanly excised wound is immediately sutured shut, if this can be done without tension (Figure 38a,b). Sutures that are tied too tight or are too closely spaced lead to necrosis by the pressure of the wound edema (Figure 39a,b). A slight gaping of the wound edges, on the other hand, has no adverse effect on the healing process or the appearance of the scar (Moberg) (Figure 40). The suturing technique (simple loop suture, Figure 41, or vertical mattress suture after Donati, Figure 42) plays only a minor role in this regard.

2. Delayed Primary Suture

If the practical limits of wound excision have been reached, then immediate closure of the wound may be followed by an infection which will ruin all our efforts. Such situations call for a delayed primary suture. The sutures are placed but not tied. The Donati suture is recommended. Further treatment follows the "delayed emergency" principle. After at most 48 hours, the decision can be made whether reduced swelling permits the sutures to be loosely tied, or whether an infection is present which must be treated according to the rules of septic hand surgery.

E. Should Antibiotics Be Used?

In all cases in which the surgeon considers primary wound closure justified, even if skin grafts are used, treatment with antibiotics is generally unnecessary.

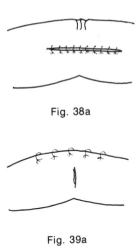

Fig. 38a

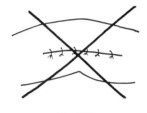

Fig. 38b

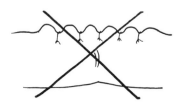
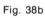

Fig. 39a

Fig. 39b

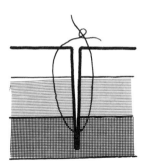

Fig. 40

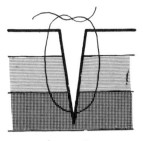

Loop suture

Fig. 41

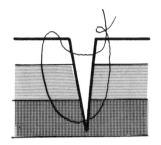

Donati suture

Fig. 42

> **Local antibiotics should never be introduced into the wound before closure!**

The consequent local tissue damage, edema formation, necrosis, etc., are greater than the antibacterial benefit.

In the delayed primary suture technique, or if the principles of delayed primary care or delayed emergency are being followed, parenteral antibiotic therapy with a broad-spectrum antibiotic is advisable.

F. Wound Closure by Plastic Measures

The transplantation of simple skin grafts, which can usually be done on an ambulatory basis, and the proper use of grafting knives and dermatomes are among the skills of any competent surgeon, including of course the hand surgeon. There are three types of grafts:

Free grafts.
Local pedicle flaps.
Distant flaps.

1. Free Grafts (Figure 43)

1) Thiersch grafts.
2) Split-skin grafts (one-half to two-thirds thickness).
3) Fat-free full-thickness grafts.
4) Reverdin grafts.

The Thiersch graft can generally be dispensed with due to its low stress resistance.

Split-skin grafts and fat-free full-thickness grafts can provide a stress-resistant covering for virtually all tissue defects, even massive ones, provided no exposed bone or unsheathed tendons are present. As the thickness of the split-skin graft decreases, it becomes increasingly prone to contracture. This must be taken into account when determining the size of the graft. The thicker the graft, the greater the demands placed on the recipient bed and the more difficult it will be for the graft to become incorporated. Once the graft is established, however, the thicker graft will be more resistant to stress than the thin graft. The split-skin graft is best taken from the thigh region by means of a dermatome (Figure 44). For small, full-thickness grafts, the most practical donor site is the inner surface of the elbow (Figure 45).

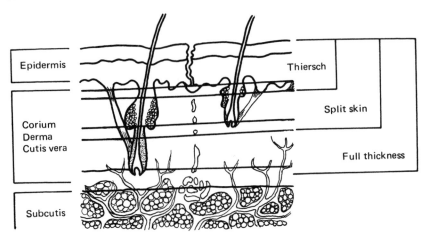

Fig. 43

The graft is sutured into the recipient bed with mersilene 5/0 under only slight tension. The free ends are tied over a mull-covered oleaginous ointment gauze topped by a piece of foam rubber for compression (Figure 46). The compression bandage is removed after 10 days. In functionally immobile or unstressed areas, open treatment with immobilization is preferred.

Reverdin grafts taken from the left hypogastrium with scissors and tweezers are among the simplest yet strongest grafts known. Their applicability in daily practice is surely better than their cosmetic reputation. They are particularly suited for repairing small defects and are held in place by a compression bandage for 10 days. They can also be sutured in place as isolated grafts. The donor sites, preferably on the left hypogastrium, can be sutured shut (Figure 47a–c) or left open.

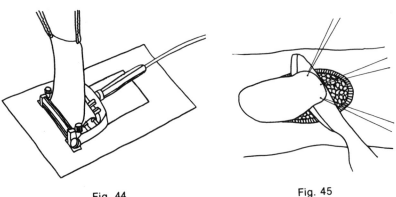

Fig. 44   Fig. 45

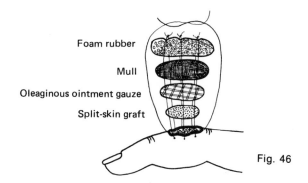

Foam rubber

Mull

Oleaginous ointment gauze

Split-skin graft

Fig. 46

2. Local Pedicle Flaps

1) Local advancement flaps (Z-plasty, visor flaps, flag flaps, rotation flaps, and V–Y advancement).
2) Volar pedicle flaps.
3) Cross-finger flaps.
4) Neurovascular flaps (Hilgenfeldt or Littler-Zrubecky).

In this type of grafting the subcutaneous fatty tissue remains attached to the flap, resulting in excellent stress resistance!

Z-plasty is not only used to correct scar contractures, but is also an excellent means of preventing them in wounds in the region of joint creases. It should be remembered that the lengthening of an area is al-

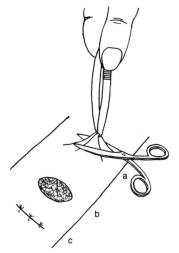

Fig. 47

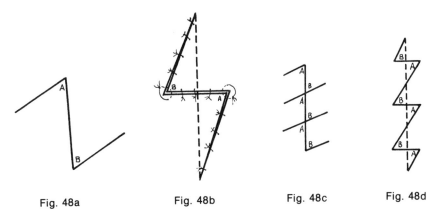

Fig. 48a   Fig. 48b   Fig. 48c   Fig. 48d

ways at the expense of its width. In the finger, this can lead to the impairment of blood flow (Figure 48a–d).

Flag flaps (Figure 49a–c) and visor flaps (Figure 50a–c) are indicated in the repair of finger stumps if the bone length must be preserved.

Rotation flaps may be indicated if a free graft cannot be used (i.e., in the joint area or over tendons and bones). They are also suited for the repair of commissures. The resultant defect is covered with a split-skin graft (Figure 51). For a lateral soft tissue defect on the finger (Bunnell), the costs are generally not justified by the gain. Here a free graft usually gives better results.

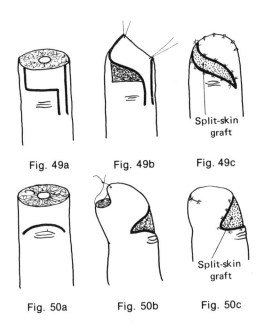

Fig. 49a   Fig. 49b   Fig. 49c

Fig. 50a   Fig. 50b   Fig. 50c

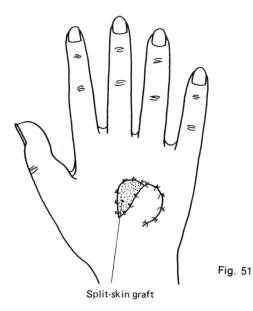

Fig. 51

Split-skin graft

The volar pedicle flap (Figure 52) is seldom used to replace a fingertip because in most cases a free graft will give the same result without the danger of contractures, especially in older patients. If the physician is considering a volar pedicle flap, he should seriously investigate whether the patient would be better off accepting the loss of a phalanx.

Cross-finger flaps for the repair of volar defects yield a skin covering that will still permit the tendons beneath it to glide (Figure 53a–c).

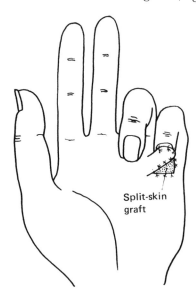

Split-skin graft

Fig. 52

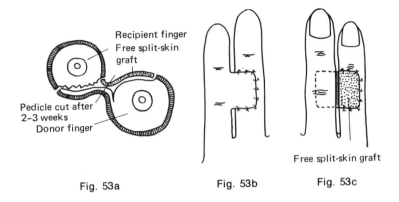

Recipient finger
Free split-skin graft

Pedicle cut after 2–3 weeks
Donor finger

Free split-skin graft

Fig. 53a   Fig. 53b   Fig. 53c

Advancement flaps (except for Z and V–Y advancements) require that the donor site be repaired with a split-skin graft. When pedicle flaps are used, the free pedicle must also be covered with split skin, since healing by granulation jeopardizes the flap by infection and contracture.

After "vascular training" by intermittent clamping of the pedicle with a rubber tube and clamp, the pedicle can be cut between the 15th and 18th day.

In all local flaps that lack a true vascular pedicle, the 2:1 ratio of flap length to pedicle width must not be exceeded lest the danger of flap necrosis arise (Figure 54).

> **The belief that pedicle flaps are more sure to take than free grafts is erroneous!**

The indications for neurovascular flaps are limited. This subject is discussed in greater detail in the chapters on Fingertip Injuries, Thumb Injuries, and Transfer Operations.

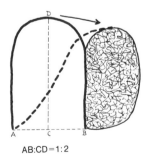

Fig. 54

AB:CD=1:2

3. Distant Flaps

This category includes bridge flaps and flat flaps from the contralateral arm, thigh, and trunk, as well as tubed pedicle flaps from the abdomen, which must be as fat free as possible while preserving the nutrient vessels. They are used to repair large-area defects on the palm and back of the hand as well as to construct secondary forms of grasp in cases of multiple finger loss. Their indications are limited, and they should be left to the experienced surgeon. The preservation of long fingers by such measures is feasible only in rare cases.

V. Correct Postoperative Procedure

1) Residual blood is removed with moist swabs to deprive bacteria of an ideal culture medium.

2) Constricting bandages must be avoided.

3) The extremity is immobilized in the position of function, or in the stress-relieved position in exceptional cases. A plaster bandage is better than a splint bandage. The flexed position, especially of the metacarpophalangeal joints, can be verified by x-ray if necessary, since the external appearance of the bandaged extremity is often deceptive.

4) The arm is elevated or suspended to promote edema drainage. This should be done with the aid of a wide, padded, full-arm wire splint, which is applied with the elbow joint flexed 100° and the inside of the elbow padded.

5) The edema is mobilized by medication.

6) Active exercise of all nonimmobilized joints from the first day on is the best prophylaxis for dystrophy. These exercises, even if they consist only of raising the arm above the horizontal, must be constantly supervised if they are to be effective. They should be performed hourly.

7) For pain relief, mild analgesics are generally sufficient. If not, the bandage must be opened and the cause of circulatory impairment determined. Infection of the wound may also be responsible for persistent pain.

> **Complaints of pain in an occlusive bandage should be taken seriously. The bandage should always be checked!**

8) Pain in the wound area that persists longer than 24 hours may indicate an incipient infection. The wound should be inspected.

9) Secondary infections during bandage changes must be avoided by aseptic precautions, especially the use of surgical masks. There is no rea-

son to open a correctly applied bandage from the 7th through 10th day as long as no complaints are voiced (see above).

10) The stitches should not be removed before the 14th day, and only after 21 days in areas subject to functional stress. A modern, non-swelling suture material permits exercise even with the stitches in place.

11) Necrotic tissues must be operatively removed promptly and the resultant defects plastically repaired as soon as possible.

Bibliography

Böhler, J.: Primäre wiederherstellende Eingriffe bei schwersten Handverletzungen. Langenbecks Arch. Chir. 292, 158 (1959).

Böhler, J.: Gewebeverpflanzungen nach Handverletzungen. Hefte Unfallheilkd. 75, 120 (1963).

Bongert, H.: Zur Behandlung komplexer, infektionsgefährdeter Handverletzungen nach dem Prinzip der Dringlichkeit mit aufgeschobener Operation *Iselin*). Hefte Unfallheilkd. 107, 242 (1971).

Buck-Gramcko, D.: Deckung von Hautdefekten an der Hand. Chir. Praxis 12, 85 (1968) 12, 263 (1968).

Buck-Gramcko, D.: Erstversorgung schwerverletzter Hände. Chir. Praxis 12, 449 (1968).

Christ, W.: Die Bedeutung erhaltener Fingernerven zur Resensibilisierung von Hauttransplantaten. Langenbecks Arch. Chir. 301, 898 (1962).

Davis, J. T.: Primary care of injuries of the hand. South. Med. J. 60, 526 (1967).

Flatt, A. E.: Minor hand injuries. J. Bone Joint Surg. 373, 80 (1957).

Gadzaly, D.: Wesentliche Vereinfachung der Spalthautverpflanzung durch Verwendung selbsthaftender Kunststoffolien. Chir. Praxis 11, 119 (1967).

Gurdin, M., Pangman, W. J.: The repair of surface defects of fingers by transdigital flaps. Plast. Reconstr. Surg. 5, 368 (1950).

Horn, J. S.: The use of full thickness hand skin flaps in the reconstruction of injured fingers. Plast. Reconstr. Surg. 7, 463 (1951).

Iselin, M.: Delayed emergency in fresh wounds of the hand. Proc. R. Soc. Med. 51, 713 (1958).

Iselin, M., Iselin, F.: Types of Z-plasty and their technical determination. J. Int. Coll. Surg. 43, 276 (1965).

Johnson, R. K., Iverson, R. E.: Cross-finger pedicle flaps in the hand. J. Bone Joint Surg. A 53, 913 (1971).

Kislov, R., Kelly, A.: Cross-finger flaps in digital injuries with notes on Kirschner-wire fixation. Plast. Reconstr. Surg. 25, 312 (1960).

Littler, J. W.: Neurovascular skin island transfer in reconstructive hand surgery. Int. Soc. Plast. Surg. 2, 175 (1960).

Marcus, G. H.: Gefahren und Fehler der kleinen Handchirurgie. Wien. Med. Wochenschr. 112, 1 (1962).

Mittelmeier, H.: Der Wundverschluß bei Handverletzungen unter besonderer Berücksichtigung primärer bzw. sekundärer plastisch-chirurgischer Maßnahmen. Chir. Plast. Reconstr. 6, 196 (1969).

Porter, R. W.: Functional assessment of transplanted skin in volar defects of the digits. A comparison between free grafts and flaps. J. Bone Joint Surg. A 50, 955 (1968).

Scharizer, E.: Die organisatorische Bedeutung der "aufgeschobenen Dringlichkeit" in der Unfallchirurgie. Hefte Unfallheilkd. 75, 146 (1963).

Schink, W.: Die Wiederherstellungschirurgie verletzter Hände. Chirurg 36, 211 (1965).

Tubiana, R.: Repair of bilateral hand mutilations. Plast. Reconstr. Surg. 44, 323 (1969).

Verdan, C.: Hautplastiken bei der Wiederherstellungschirurgie der verletzten Hand. Langenbecks Arch. Chir. 299, 69 (1961).

Verdan, C.: Basic principles in surgery of the hand. Surg. Clin. North Am. 47, 355 (1967).

Zrubecky, G.: Derzeitige Grenzen bei der planmäßigen Versorgung schwerer Handverletzungen. Hefte Unfallheilkd. 83 (1965).

Amputations

The primary function of the hand is the grasping and holding of objects. It does so with an action similar to the jaws of a pliers, with four three-membered digits opposed by a single thumb. The interaction of these elements must be so precise that even tiny objects can be grasped. They must also have a spread sufficient to grasp bulky objects as well. The natural forms of grasp derive from the various ways in which the two basic elements of grasp (fingers and thumb) interact. We distinguish between the precision or pinch grip, the key grip, the gross or power grip, and the hook grip (Figures 5–8). The preservation of these primary forms of grasp is the foremost goal of the treatment of hand injuries. If necessary, an attempt is made to create secondary forms of grasp.

Despite the progress made in plastic and reparative surgery, primary and secondary amputations cannot always be avoided. In the case of upper extremity amputations, however, it should always be remembered that a prosthesis can never even come close to imitating the natural functions in a satisfactory manner, due mainly to the absence of sensation. Thus, when amputation is unavoidable, the operation must be carefully planned so as to preserve as much functionally worthwhile natural tissue as possible. Every part of a finger whose function can be preserved will improve the grasping ability of an injured hand, even if it enables only secondary forms of grasp to be developed spontaneously or by operative means. The thumb, as the only opponent of the long fingers, is especially important in this regard. If removal of several fingers including the thumb is unavoidable, it may be possible to surgically construct a thumb from an involved finger or finger remnant (Figure 55).

If the attending surgeon is lacking in experience, the evaluation and operation should be left to a colleague who possesses the necessary skills. In view of the prospects opened up by the "emergency with delayed operation" and "delayed primary care" techniques discussed earlier, an ap-

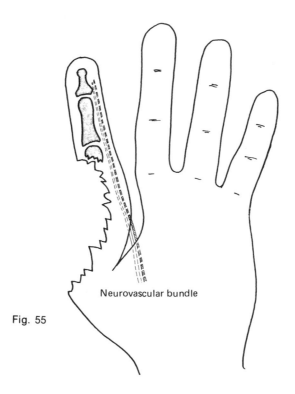

Neurovascular bundle

Fig. 55

parent time loss of many hours is insignificant compared with the potential benefits to the patient. *An absolute indication for amputation is present only if the blood supply has been completely suspended in a part and restoration of the vascular system is impossible.* An intact artery on the volar side is sufficient to nourish a finger, and a dorsal artery is adequate for the thumb. A dorsal artery can also nourish a proximal phalanx stump. The impossibility of skin closure or the destruction of joints, tendons, or nerves alone should never be sufficient grounds for amputation. Remember the following points:

Skin grafts can be used to effect primary closure.
Fingers that are stiffened in the articular position of function are far from useless.
Tendon transfers and, in case of nerve damage, motor and sensory transfers can be employed.
Severed members can, under favorable conditions, be replanted by microsurgical techniques.

Of course, the costs of restorative surgery should be outweighed by its potential benefits, taking into account the age, occupation, and intelligence of the patient. The decision to amputate will thus be easier in the case of a single, severely damaged long finger than in the case of several fingers with similar injuries. There is a danger of wanting to "save too much." In case of doubt, however, *primary* preservation by wound closure (using simple skin grafts if necessary) and perhaps *secondary* amputation are preferable to *primary* amputation. In the final analysis, only experience will help the surgeon to assess the situation correctly, and every surgeon must gain that for himself.

During routine primary care of an amputation, every effort must be made to preserve remaining functions while avoiding rash measures that might jeopardize the restoration of substitute functions.

Of practical importance in this regard is the problem of the prosthetic care of hand amputees. With the development of pneumatically and bioelectrically controlled gripping devices, modern prosthetics have made a valuable contribution to vocational and social rehabilitation. However, the benefits of these devices have so far been reserved for a relatively small circle of select amputees whose wish for a prosthesis is based on more than just the desire to conceal the loss of an extremity: the wish for vocational rehabilitation, combined with the will to master the prosthesis problem and the intelligence to handle this "miracle of technology." These are essentially the requirements for any rehabilitation.

For the overwhelming majority of cases, a well-formed stump with normal sensation is more valuable than an insensible prosthesis and is often even a prerequisite for such a device.

During the planning of an operation, the following general points must be considered to properly care for the various anatomical structures.

I. Care of the Skin

A scar that adheres to bone or tendon may limit the motion of a joint or even lead to the stiffening of an entire finger. If this scar crosses the hand lines and especially joint creases at a right angle, contractures often result. Nerves surrounded by scar tissue lose a portion of their function, and nerve stumps that terminate in the scar cause constant discomfort and can make a stump functionally useless. Thin skin which tightly covers a bone stump or even secondary epithelium on a stump is constantly susceptible to damage. Thus, a *tension-free* closure with good skin must be achieved on the stump, with no functionally important structures lying in the scar area (Figure 56a–c).

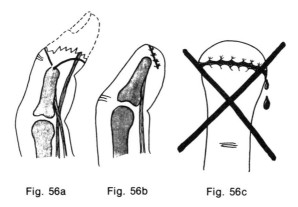

Fig. 56a   Fig. 56b   Fig. 56c

Ideally, the amputation scar should lie on the dorsal side. A higher amputation is not justified on this account, however. Instead, the tip of the stump can be covered with laterally or dorsally pedicled flaps, provided they consist of well-nourished, stress-resistant skin (Figure 57a,b). When the preservation of an important function is at stake, skin grafts are indicated. Of course the use of abdominal pedicle flaps to preserve a finger is advisable only in exceptional cases, especially on the thumb.

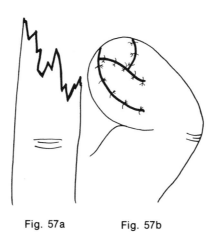

Fig. 57a   Fig. 57b

II. Care of the Bones

If pinching instruments (Luer or Lister) are used to cut the bone, splintering usually occurs. Better results are obtained with a small saw. Fractures of unamputated parts of the extremity require accurate reduction and fixation in order to avoid malunions and the accompanying impairment of function.

III. Care of the Tendons

> **The traditional practice of uniting the tendons over the bone stump is both unnecessary and undesirable in the case of the fingers.**

Tendons that are united over a finger stump are primarily motors for the amputated portion of the finger, rather than the remaining part. When they are joined, they impair the mobility of both the stump and the remaining fingers, since the tendinous junctions of the extensor tendons and the origin of the long flexor tendons from a common muscle package limit the excursion of all the tendons. Even the "independent" index finger cannot be fully flexed while another long finger is fixed in extension. The nonphysiological fixation of the long tendons of a finger must therefore be avoided. Instead, they should be shortened as much as possible and then allowed to retract palmarward. Only in central amputations is fixation of the antagonists desirable in order to preserve muscle length, tone, and relief for possible prosthetic measures.

IV. Care of the Neurovascular Bundles

The neurovascular bundles of the fingers are not always easy to find, but must be located for two reasons:

1) The nerve must be shortened to prevent adherence of its terminal neuroma to the scar.
2) Ligature of the vessels is desirable (Figure 58a,b).

To be sure, bleeding from a digital artery usually stops by itself, but even slight secondary bleeding can cause a hematoma and thus lead to circulatory disorders and granulation healing at the stump. Ligatures in the finger are made with catgut 6/0. More proximal vessels require a stronger suture material, which should still be as thin as possible. The resultant foreign body reaction is mild and appears to be the lesser evil.

The amputation procedure for the various parts of the hand is dictated by local anatomical conditions, which will be described below in more detail. A separate chapter is devoted to the care of fingertip injuries due to the special importance of this zone for grasping.

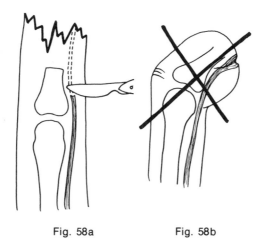

Fig. 58a   Fig. 58b

V. Thumb Amputations

A general rule is that an effort must be made to preserve every millimeter of bone length possible by plastic measures. The mobility of the
basal and terminal joints need not be taken into consideration. Even a
shortened, stiff thumb can fully exercise its function of opposition. Preservation of the base of the first metacarpal bone and thus of the saddle
joint is important with regard to operative reconstruction of the thumb,
which may prove necessary and is almost always possible.

VI. Amputation at the Middle Phalanx
of the Long Fingers

Extension in the middle joint is accomplished chiefly by the middle
slip of the extensor apparatus. If its insertion at the base of the middle
phalanx can be preserved, extension will be unimpaired. The insertions
of the two slips of the superficial flexor of the finger radiate far into the
periosteum of the middle phalanx. If a strong enough portion of one or
preferably both insertions can be preserved, flexion of the middle joint
will be ensured (Figure 59a–c). Otherwise it is better to remove the middle phalanx, in which case the head of the proximal phalanx is freed of
cartilage and rounded. In each case the unneeded tendons of the finger
flexors are pulled forward and cut so that they retract (Figure 60a,b).

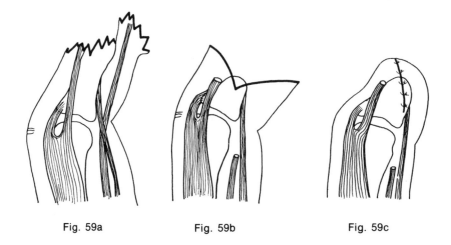

Fig. 59a   Fig. 59b   Fig. 59c

VII. Amputation at the Basal Phalanx of the Long Fingers

Amputation even very near the base of the basal phalanx is preferable to exarticulation. Even a short stump still plays an important role in generating force during the power grip, even if it serves no purpose other than to maintain the width of the hand. Such an arrangement is admittedly unattractive, but for manual laborers at least, function ranks above appearance. The proximal phalanx of the little finger is especially valuable in this respect. It must be remembered during the amputation that extension in the basal joint is accomplished by part of the middle slip (extensor communis) of the extensor apparatus, which is inserted dor-

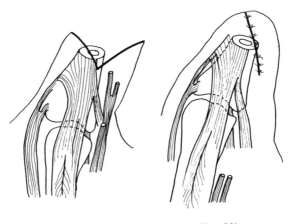

Fig. 60a   Fig. 60b

sally into the base of the proximal phalanx, whereas the small hand muscles bring about flexion while joined to the extensor aponeurosis (Figure 60a,b). Accordingly, these tendons must remain intact while the long flexors are shortened.

VIII. Exarticulation of One or More Fingers

If the complete removal of one or more fingers appears unavoidable, every effort must be made to leave behind a hand remnant that can still produce primary or secondary forms of grasp; the exact form of the remnant depends on the individual needs of the patient. In general, the primary considerations are not cosmetic. The incisions are shown in Figure 61.

When the third or fourth finger is removed, the concurrent removal of the distal third of the associated metacarpal is permitted in the case of "white collar" and other nonmanual workers (Adelmann, 1888). This brings about a cosmetic narrowing of the hand, and the angulation of the adjacent fingers and thus their functional impairment is smaller than if the head of the metacarpal were left intact (Figure 62). If both fingers must be amputated, simple exarticulation is recommended for manual workers in order to preserve at least the width of the remaining power grip. In this case the heads of the associated metacarpals are simply freed of cartilage and rounded (Figure 63).

> **An Adelmann hand is unsuited for heavy labor.**

The same applies to removal of the second through fourth fingers.

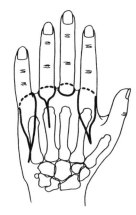

Fig. 61

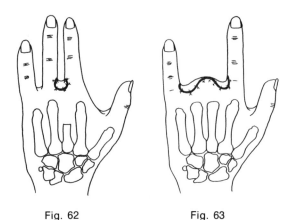

Fig. 62   Fig. 63

However, not all patients are capable of forming a strong secondary pinch grip between the thumb and little finger. Rotational osteotomy may be the answer in such cases. It is best done at the shaft of the fifth metacarpal near its base, bringing the little finger in opposition to the thumb. Fixation is accomplished with Kirschner wires. To speed healing of the bone, a chip graft from a phalanx to be amputated can be pinned in during primary care, or a graft from the proximal ulna can be used at secondary operation (Figure 64a,b).

In order to obtain at least secondary forms of grasp for severely injured hands, an attempt should be made to preserve as many damaged fingers as possible. Assuming an adequate blood supply, there are two possible techniques for accomplishing this besides skin grafting: First, a defect pseudarthrosis can be left until it is later united by means of an autologous bone graft (Figure 147). Second, primary shortening of the finger, possibly combined with arthrodesis, may make amputation un-

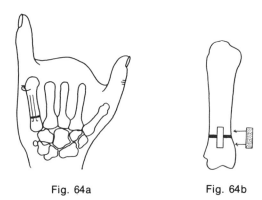

Fig. 64a   Fig. 64b

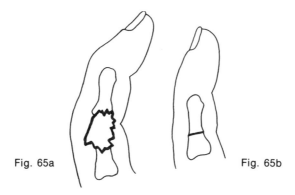

Fig. 65a   Fig. 65b

necessary (Figure 65a,b). Sometimes a portion of the base of the proximal phalanx of the index finger can be retained along with a stiffened basal joint. The result is a rigid strut which, though cosmetically unappealing, may greatly aid the patient in executing the key grip.

If the index finger must be removed, the concurrent oblique resection of the associated metacarpal in the central third of its shaft is advised (especially for manual laborers). Interaction between the thumb and the other fingers is facilitated by this measure and by transferring the first interosseous to the third finger (Figure 66).

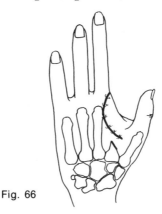

Fig. 66

The procedure is essentially the same for removal of the index and middle finger; the only difference is that the third metacarpal is obliquely resected at a more distal point (Figure 67) in order to preserve the adductability of the thumb by sparing the muscle origin.

Conditions are somewhat different at the fifth finger. In this case removal of the entire ray is the most cosmetic solution (Figure 68). For the manual worker, of course, it might be better to retain the fifth metacarpal so as to maintain a full palm width for gripping tools.

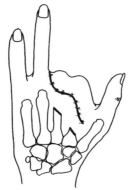

Fig. 67

The complete loss of all four long fingers naturally makes all forms of grasp impossible, but the smooth amputation of all the long fingers at the level of the basal joint is an extremely rare occurrence. In most cases there are some flaps of skin left on the volar side, perhaps still with sensation. These flaps of skin must be carefully preserved in their entirety. One should not hesitate to allow a flaccid sack of soft tissue to heal or allow volar sensory skin to take on the dorsal side by extension of the wound. The experienced surgeon may later be able to use such tissue to construct a rudimentary, immobile, yet sensible digit that is useful in grasping. This is made easier if, during primary care, an otherwise useless phalanx devoid of its soft tissues is buried beneath the thoracic skin of the contralateral side.

The same is true for the concurrent loss of the thumb. It should be noted in passing that the nourished skin of a useless finger is ideal for use in primary wound closure or as a replacement for poor scar tissue (Figure 69a,b).

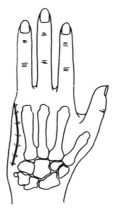

Fig. 68

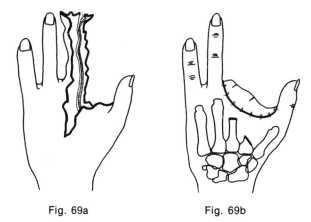

Fig. 69a   Fig. 69b

Even if all the fingers are lost, it will at least be possible to restore a secondary form of grasp by creating a prehensile hand remnant. For this purpose a cleft is formed between the first and second metacarpals. The circumstances will determine whether this should be done by simple Z-plasty (Figure 70a–c) or by forming a flap by the Kreuz method (Figure 71). Even if the opposable surfaces of the remnant must be covered with free grafts and are thus devoid of sensation, the operation is worthwhile in view of the severity of the functional losses. This formation of a prehensile cleft, or deepening of a cleft if the thumb is only partially lost, requires that the nerves in the region of the cleft be carefully preserved. The distal portion of the adductor muscle of the thumb, which extends toward the third metacarpal, is notched in order to achieve the necessary depth (Figure 72). It is important for the function of the mobile part of the remnant that the short flexor of the thumb be preserved.

Finally, in cases of total bilateral finger loss, there is still the possibility of constructing "metacarpal fingers."

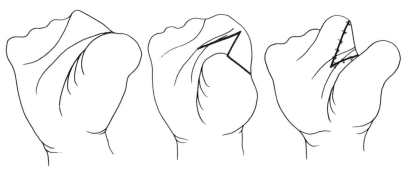

Fig. 70a   Fig. 70b   Fig. 70c

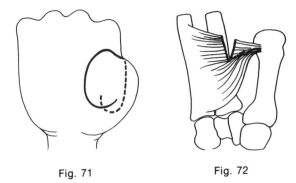

Fig. 71   Fig. 72

The examples given are intended to show how complex the problems of preserving or restoring a grasp function are in cases of finger loss. The fate of a severely injured hand is usually decided during the primary care phase. The *first* surgeon must therefore decide what may be sacrificed and what must be preserved so as to maximize the chances for the subsequent correction of faulty grasps, improvement of a hand remnant, or production of secondary forms of grasp.

IX. Carpometacarpal Amputation

Even the short stump left by carpometacarpal amputation is more valuable than an insensible prosthesis. It is especially important that the stump be provided with a good covering of skin and soft tissue so that it can be used to push, pull, and hold large objects. The thenar and hypothenar muscles are therefore used to pad the stump.

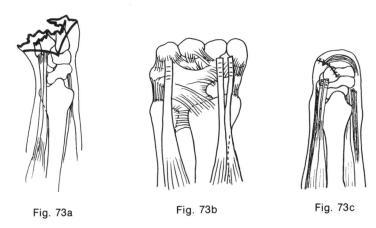

Fig. 73a   Fig. 73b   Fig. 73c

The nerves are dealt with in the usual manner. The finger tendons are shortened and allowed to retract. To improve remaining functions, an attempt must be made to obtain mobility in the radiocarpal joint. Thus if the flexors and extensors of the wrist have lost their insertions, they are reinserted into the carpal bones after the cortical substance is roughened (Figure 73a–c). During closure of the soft tissues, care should be taken that the suture of the deeper soft tissues is in a different plane from the cutaneous suture because the stump covering has a tendency to shift.

X. Exarticulation at the Wrist and Forearm Amputations

At the wrist and distal half of the forearm, the stump cannot be padded with muscle for anatomical reasons. It is important, therefore, that the bone be carefully rounded and the stump covered with good skin. The tendon stumps are fixed to the bone to preserve the forearm relief with a view toward prosthetic care. In bilateral amputees, this is essential for producing a Krukenberg hand (Figures 74a–c, 75a–c).

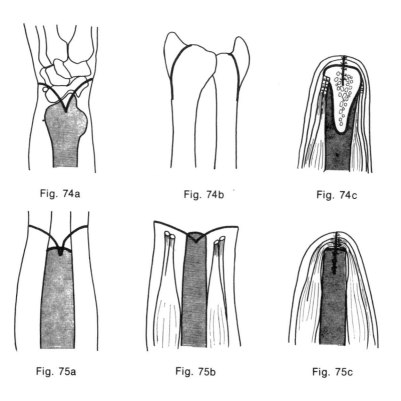

Fig. 74a   Fig. 74b   Fig. 74c

Fig. 75a   Fig. 75b   Fig. 75c

XI. Replantation of Severed Members

Increasingly, severe injuries of the upper extremity are raising the question of restoration by vascular and neural anastomosis. Microsurgery has doubtlessly opened up new possibilities in this regard. If the technical and personal facilities for such a procedure are available or can be made available at short notice, it is worth a try.

A. Indications for Replantation

1) All central amputations.
2) Amputation of the thumb.
3) Amputation of several long fingers.

B. Prognosis of Replantation

Smooth amputations by a sharp trauma offer the best prospects for replantation. Crushing amputations have a poorer prognosis. Avulsions are problematic from the outset.

C. Treatment of Amputation Stump

1) No debridement.
2) No hemostasis.
3) Compression bandage only.

D. Treatment of Amputated Member

1) No debridement.
2) No perfusion.
3) Waterproof packing (plastic bag).
4) Dry cooling to about 4°C (the plastic bag with the amputated member is packed in ice in a second plastic bag).

Freezing of the member or contact with melted ice must be avoided.

The maximum survival time of the amputated member before replantation (Owen) is as follows:

Arm: 10 hours.
Hand: 12 hours.
Finger: 24 hours.

Bibliography

Balas, P., et al.: The present status of replantation of amputated extremities. Vasc. Surg. 4, 190 (1970).

Burkhalter, W. E., Mayfield, G., Carmona, L. S.: The upper-extremity amputee: Early and immediate postsurgical prosthetic fitting. J. Bone Joint Surg. A 58, 46 (1976).

Chase, R. A.: Functional levels of amputation in the hand. Surg. Clin. North Am. 40, 287 (1960).

Chase, R. A.: The severely injured upper limb. To amputate or reconstruct, that is the question. Arch. Surg. 100, 382 (1970).

Herndon, J. H., Eaton, R. G., Littler, J. W.: Management of painful neuromas in the hand. J. Bone Joint Surg. A 58, 369 (1976).

Kuhn, G. G.: Die prothetische Versorgung der Hand. Hefte Unfallheilkd. 75, 93 (1963).

Malt, R. A., McKhann, C. F.: Replantation of severed arms. JAMA 189, 716 (1964).

Millesi, H., Meissl, G., Berger, A.: The interfascicular nerve grafting of the median and ulnar nerves. J. Bone Joint Surg. A 54, 727 (1972).

Millesi, H., Meissl, G., Berger, A.: Further experience with interfascicular grafting of the median, ulnar and radial nerves. J. Bone Joint Surg. A 58, 209 (1976).

Owen, E. R.: Replantation abgetrennter Gliedmassen. Langenbecks Arch. Chir. 339, 613 (1975).

Peacock, E. E., Jr.: Metacarpal transfer following amputation of a central digit. Plast. Reconstr. Surg. 29, 345 (1962).

Pieper, W.: Fingererhaltung durch operative Gelenkversteifung in Funktionsstellung. Langenbecks Arch. Chir. 299, 126 (1961).

Rahmel, R.: Grenzen der Erhaltung von Fingern bei schweren Verletzungen. Chir. Praxis 12, 275 (1968).

Schmidt-Tintemann, N., et al.: Replantation abgetrennter Finger, Daumen und Hände durch Mikrochirurgie. Dtsch. Ärztebl. 1367 (1976). .

Simon, P.: Die Metaphalangisation. Z. Orthop. 97, 551 (1963).

Streli, R.: Zur Technik der Fingerarthrodese. Chir. Praxis 1, 327 (1957).

Takayuki, J., et al.: Factors necessary for successful replantation of upper extremities. Ann. Surg. 165, 225 (1967).

Tooms, R. E.: Amputation surgery in the upper extremity. Orthop. Clin. North Am. 3, 383 (1972).

Williams, G. R., et al.: Replantation of amputated extremities. Ann. Surg. 163, 788 (1966).

Fingertip Injuries

The fingertips are sense organs that tell us the temperature, shape, and texture of all objects with which they come into contact. The ability for spatial comprehension, or tactile gnosis, is resident in the tips of the fingers. The nail bed, also rich in nerve end organs, and the nail, which acts as a support for the soft volar tissues, serve as mediators of cutaneous sensation. Finally, the bone forms the stable axis of the fingertip. The bone, bulb, and nail thus comprise a functional unit. Its injury or destruction may make it impossible to perform an otherwise simple act.

Despite this fact, fingertip injuries are usually dismissed as trivial. If we realize the differentiated structures that are affected, however, it becomes clear that these "trivial" injuries call for thoughtful treatment in order to achieve satisfactory functional and cosmetic results. What surgeon, after all, could do without his fingertip sensation! The goal of the treatment must be as complete an anatomical restoration as possible, with special attention given to the preservation or restoration of cutaneous sensation.

I. Subungual Hematoma

Blood may collect beneath the nail as the result of a wound of the nail bed or bleeding into the loose tissue in the region of the lunula, the crescentic light area at the nail base. The pressure of the hematoma causes intense throbbing pains, which require the relief of pressure by trepanation of the nail (Figure 76) or, if necessary, its removal. Trepanation, which consists of drilling a small hole *distal* to the lunula, does afford some relief of pain but raises the danger of infection of the subungual space, which often requires extensive surgical measures as well as secondary removal of the nail. On the other hand, simple removal of the

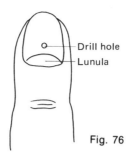

Fig. 76

nail—done by lifting with a dissector, closed scissors, or, preferably, nail forceps without a preliminary longitudinal cut, care being taken to preserve the bed, lunula, and matrix—also alleviates the pain but does not make it possible to control scar formation in the region of the nail bed. Many a nail deformity results from excessive granulation and hypertrophic scars in the nail bed. Because removal of the nail requires anesthesia anyway, it takes little additional time to clean the nail, adapt the nail bed wound by suturing with catgut 4/0, and biologically resplint the bed with the nail. In this procedure the root of the nail must be pushed back under the proximal nail fold, where it is fixed by suturing with mersilene 4/0 (Figure 77). If, as often happens, the nail hangs on its cuticle when lifted, the procedure is still the same. The change of bandage after 10 days is painless. By then the nail is usually so firmly adherent that the sutures can be removed. After 6 weeks at most, the replanted nail will be expelled by the new nail.

II. Loss of the Nail

Neumann has reported good results with homeoplastic preserved nails. This technique is promising with regard to the undisturbed re-

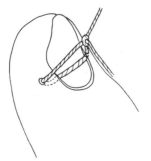

Fig. 77

growth of the nail. "Bank nails" of this type are not always available, however, and simple bandaging with an oleaginous ointment gauze will usually have to do. It is unlikely that the transplantation of toenails would ever be warranted.

III. Nail Deformities

The aesthetic results of efforts to treat the injured fingernail are not always perfect. However, considering that the absence of the nail means a loss of fingertip sensitivity, and that its presence often appears to be more valuable than full fingertip sensation, such malformations as furrows, fissures, hour-glass deformities, and even certain forms of claw nail should be tolerated, and dissatisfied patients should be informed of the importance of the nail. Women with cosmetically unappealing nail deformities can lengthen and beautify their nails by applying a plastic substance that hardens in the air. Such products are offered by the cosmetic industry.

Split nails result from adhesions between the nail matrix and fold. They are sometimes amenable to treatment if, after the split nail is removed, recurrence of the adhesions is prevented by constant probing until the new nail has grown in. This condition offers yet another indication for the "bank nail."

Because a scar-damaged matrix cannot be replaced, its complete extirpation may sometimes be necessary in order to prevent the regrowth of nail from it. In some cases it is necessary to replace the vulnerable secondary epithelium of the nail bed with a more resistant graft. Then artificial stick-on nails, also available commercially, can be worn for cosmetic reasons when needed. Overlooked matrix remnants produce tiny, sharp, irritating nail splinters which require a second operation for complete extirpation of the matrix.

IV. Fractures of the Distal Phalanx

These fractures are usually combined with injuries of the nail and nail bed. Closed fractures of the nail insertion themselves require no special treatment. However, they are extremely painful in the beginning, and a protective plaster splint is advised for a few days. In the case of open comminuted fractures, the small fragments are removed to prevent sequestration. After the larger fragments are reduced, the edges of the bed wound are adapted with catgut 4/0. Finally, the often avulsed matrix

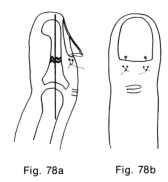

Fig. 78a   Fig. 78b

must again be fixed beneath the nail fold (Nichols; Figure 78a,b). If the nail is still present, it is replanted. It provides an excellent splint for the fracture fragments and also protects the wound surface of the nail bed. The transverse fracture of the distal phalanx is fixed for 4 weeks with percutaneous drill wire (0.8–1.0 mm in diameter), with temporary arthrodesis of the terminal joint in slight flexion if necessary to improve stability (Figure 78a).

A fine punctural incision is made. Drill wire is introduced until contact with bone is made. The wire must be drilled in parallel to the nail bed. Remember that the bone lies just below the nail bed. The use of a 5- to 6-cm length of wire is sufficient; a longer wire could not be guided with precision. The end of the wire is snipped off below skin level and buried. The drilling speed must be high enough to ensure smooth passage of the wire, not so high as to cause thermal injury. Irrigation with physiological saline is mandatory. Fractures of the distal phalanx which remain ununited generally require no special treatment as long as the nail provides the necessary stability.

Epiphyseal fractures in the child must be carefully reduced and immobilized with a splint for 3 weeks. If this treatment is inadequate, drill wire osteosynthesis may be undertaken with no fear of adverse consequences.

V. Fingertip Hematoma in the Child

This is a special form of childhood injury. Undetected and infected, it will have adverse consequences, as pointed out by Recht. Infected hematomas must be promptly opened by a half-frogmouth incision before the infection spreads to the bone. Closed fingertip injuries in children must thus be carefully inspected, because in most children the condition goes undetected until osteomyelitis of the distal phalanx causes severe pain.

VI. Defect Wounds

Primary healing of the wound by surgical measures is most desirable. All possibilities for restoring cutaneous sensation, and thus fingertip sensation, must be exhausted if there is to be a reasonable prospect of success.

Several approaches can be taken:

1) Primary suture of the wound, with a shortening of the bone if necessary.
2) Secondary amputation.
3) Free grafts.
4) Local pedicle flaps.
5) Sensory transfers.
6) Distant flaps.

A fingertip wound should not be allowed to heal by granulation and thus become covered by an inferior integument of secondary epithelium, unless the wound is an abrasion or a very small, superficial tissue defect that can be treated with an oleaginous gauze dressing. Although Kleinert believes that defects up to 1 cm in diameter can be tolerated, this estimate seems somewhat high. We believe, along with other authors, that the results of modern hand surgery make the operative care of such wounds advisable.

A. Primary Suture

The primary suture is feasible only if it can be placed without tension. With a wedge-shaped wound excision, it is usually successful only if the bone is shortened slightly (Figure 79a–c).

B. Secondary Amputation

Secondary amputation in cases of partial finger loss according to zur Verth's scheme, i.e., in an injury of the distal phalanx below the head of the middle phalanx, in no way represents the optimal therapeutic technique. It should be reserved only for cases in which the fingertip remnant is so small that the flexor and extensor have lost their reacting organ. In such cases the profundus tendon is pulled as far forward as possible and clipped. It then retracts by itself into the palm and will not

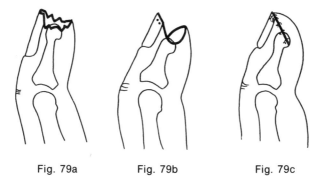

Fig. 79a   Fig. 79b   Fig. 79c

interfere with the function of the superficial tendon. If the tendon insertions are intact, secondary amputation may be limited to part of the fingertip and may even leave parts of the nail behind (Figure 80a–c). An
important consideration in determining the length of any finger stump,
and especially the distal phalanx stump, is that it should be able to be
well covered with soft tissue. This must be taken into account when the
bone is shortened. Too much soft tissue interferes with grasp (Figure
81a–c).

Where the long fingers are concerned, a well-padded stump is better,
despite the loss of length, than poor scar conditions or an insensible
graft on a finger of normal length.

Even stumps with a good covering of soft tissue are often rendered
useless by painful neuromas, which can promote circulatory disorders
not only in the injured finger, but also in the hand as a whole. Neuroma
carriers sometimes become "neuroma patients," who can rarely be
helped by surgical measures. To prevent this, the nerve stumps are located *during primary care* and shortened by 4–6 mm, so that they retract

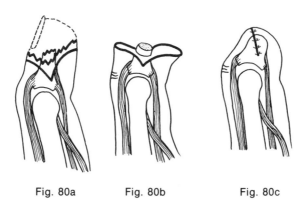

Fig. 80a   Fig. 80b   Fig. 80c

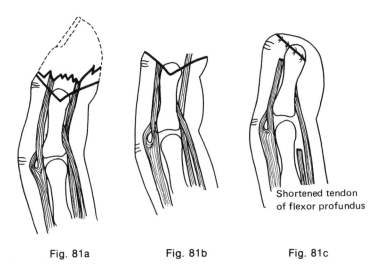

Fig. 81a   Fig. 81b   Fig. 81c

into the loose fat and can no longer adhere to the scar. The fascicles can
be clearly distinguished with the naked eye from the vessels by examining the cross section of the fiber. If the stump is made useless by
neuromas, which can usually be easily felt as painful nodules in the scar
area, the nerve stumps must be examined without delay. They are located and sufficiently shortened and, if necessary, displaced into the
bone.

A stump that is poorly covered with soft tissue and has a deficient
blood supply requires secondary amputation in any case, to the extent
that a tension-free covering with well-perfused, scar-free skin can be
achieved.

Stump corrections are among the most commonplace operations in
hand surgery. In view of the fact that such an operation results in an
average of 3 weeks additional lost work time for the patient, it is important that the stump be correctly formed the first time.

C. Free Grafts

Grafts suitable for use on the fingertip are Reverdin grafts (Figure
47a–c) and fat-free full-thickness grafts (Figure 45). Only these grafts
can withstand the considerable stresses placed on the grasping surfaces
of the fingers. Reverdin grafts should be reserved for small defects, however, because they are prone to troublesome cicatrization even with careful adaptation at the edges of the graft.

A disadvantage of both grafts is their inability to restore tactile gnosis.
Within a few months, however, these grafts are likely to develop a pro-

tective sensation which will protect against gross injuries, so the finger is far from functionally useless. This must be remembered, especially in the case of multiple finger injuries. The transplantation of a toe tip is an unnecessary and somewhat risky procedure.

In terms of function, free skin grafts may leave much to be desired, especially when used on the fingertips. However, for only a slight investment of operative and postoperative care, primary healing is achieved with no loss of finger length. Even the less experienced surgeon will have no difficulties in achieving good results. Thus the free graft is particularly suited for ambulatory care.

D. Local Pedicle Flaps

Closure of the wound by the use of local pedicle flaps presents greater technical difficulties than do free grafts. The physician must decide on a case-by-case basis which type of flap the patient requires—advancement flaps (Geissendorfer, Kutler, Tranquilli-Leali), visor flaps (Bunnell, de Jong, Klapp; Figure 50a–c), or local pedicle flaps from the dorsum (Villain; Figure 49a–c), thenar and palm (J. Boehler, Gatewood, Jones; Figure 52), or an adjacent finger (Cronin, Gurdin, Iselin, Pangman, Tempest; Figure 53a–c). These flaps can produce cosmetically sound fingertips or stump ties with excellent stress-bearing properties and good pain sensation, if not full tactile gnosis.

When visor and flag flaps are used, the donor area must be repaired with a free graft. Flaps from an adjacent finger or the palm, moreover, require that the free pedicle be covered with a Thiersch graft in order to prevent granulation. The operative investment is therefore relatively large. If healing of the wound is impaired, the function of the entire hand is jeopardized. Section of the pedicle and the final extension of the flap can generally be accomplished during the third week. Before then,

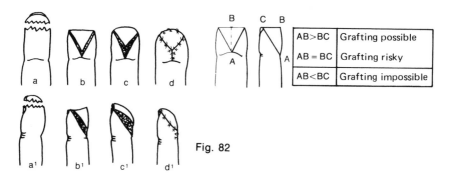

AB>BC	Grafting possible
AB = BC	Grafting risky
AB<BC	Grafting impossible

Fig. 82

the pedicle should be clamped off to make sure the flap has become attached to the recipient bed.

V–Y advancement by the Tranquilli-Leali method appears to be the procedure of choice, provided the extent of the fingertip amputation makes its use possible (Figure 82). The V-shaped incision is always made such that the tip of the V extends to the flexion crease of the terminal joint, even if it may appear that a smaller flap would do. The incision is deepened until small globules of fatty tissue appear. If difficulties arise during distal advancement of the flap, mobilization of the vessel-poor center of the ventral cusp and at the distal end of the incisions can be undertaken without endangering sensation. Often the injury is accompanied by considerable swelling of the fingertip, making grafting questionable. It is advisable in such cases to resort to the delayed primary suture technique, whereby the sutures initially placed are drawn tight after the swelling has subsided (usually after 48 hours). In some cases the nails will continue their growth in an hourglass fashion as a result of scar tension, especially whenever the experienced surgeon perceives an indication for dermoplasty even in cases for which amputation must be considered. It is unlikely that functional losses will occur in such cases, as our own follow-up studies have shown. Of course, the faulty practice of this method will end in flap necrosis and infection.

This form of finger-pad grafting provides restoration of cutaneous sensation on the fingertip as well as a skin covering. The flap can, in fact, be classified as neurovascular, an advantage seldom shared by visor flaps or flag flaps taken from the palm and adjacent fingers due to section of the pedicle.

One should thus be very hesitant to use grafts on the fingertips that offer little prospect of restoring tactile gnosis. In consideration of vocational demands, we recommend secondary amputation in such cases and would limit length-preserving surgery to multiple finger injuries in which it is important to preserve natural forms of grasp or to construct secondary forms.

The applications of pedicle flaps from the palm or adjacent fingers are further limited to the extent that elderly persons, rheumatic patients, and persons with "sausage fingers" should be excluded from treatment. In such persons there is a considerable danger of stiffening of the involved finger joints.

E. Sensory Transfers

A lost finger bulb can be repaired with a neurovascular island flap (Littler-Zrubecky), a special type of local pedicle flap that is based on Hilgenfeldt's principle of interdigital sensory transfer. It is well to place much stricter limits on the indications for this operation than do many surgeons, however.

This procedure should be reserved for cases in which the "functionally critical zones" of the soft tissue of fingers one through three are destroyed, while the bone length remains complete. We shall return to these flaps in later discussions of thumb injuries and surgical reconstruction.

F. Distant Flaps

In general, distant flaps from the arm, leg, or torso are not well suited functionally for fingertip injuries. An exception is the complete skeletization of the thumb.

Rejection of the graft or flap necrosis occasionally occurs in any form of dermoplasty. In these cases, which fortunately are rare, one should not throw up one's hands, but must try to bring about primary healing by excising the necrotic tissue and regrafting the wound. The beginner should note that free skin grafts are technically simpler and no more prone to necrosis than pedicle flaps.

The procedure selected for a particular case will be determined on the one hand by the extent of the injury, the occupation, age, sex, and intelligence, of the patient, and cosmetic considerations. On the other hand, the indication for this or any other method will depend in large measure on the experience of the surgeon, who, incidentally, should never succumb to the temptation of wanting to "save too much." If functionally critical zones of the hand have been largely restored in terms of anatomical shape but are deprived of cutaneous sensation, the patient is exposed to the danger of reinjury.

The following procedure is therefore recommended:

1)   In injuries of a long finger, the bulb is provided with a sensible cover by V–Y advancement of the Tranquilli-Leali type; otherwise the fingertip is amputated to produce a stress-resistant stump. If the patient objects to this form of treatment, he is informed of the possible adverse consequences of an insensible fingertip. The cover is then produced by free grafting.

2)   Small defects in areas of little functional importance are covered with fat-free full-thickness grafts. An attempt is made to fill the defect completely with *one* Reverdin graft.

3)   In multiple finger injuries the procedure is determined by the individual needs of the patient. It is here that fingers with no cutaneous sensation must sometimes be preserved in order to create secondary

forms of grasp. These situations are generally the domain of the local pedicle flaps in their various forms, but the free graft is sometimes called for. The care of these injuries should therefore be left to the experienced surgeon.

VII. Extensor Tendon Injuries of the Distal Phalanx

The most frequent cause of extensor tendon injuries, aside from sharp divisions, is a blow to the slightly flexed finger, resulting in the closed avulsion of the extensor aponeurosis at the fingertip, with or without bone involvement.

A. Diagnosis

The terminal joint is flexed and cannot be actively extended.

B. Differential Diagnosis

Swan-neck deformity occurs in rupture of the volar fibrocartilage of the middle joint, whereby the terminal joint is in flexion and the middle joint in hyperextension. During passive flexion of the middle joint, the terminal joint can be fully extended.

C. Treatment

The treatment depends on the type of injury:

1. Open Division of Extensor Tendon
   without Bone Involvement

Wound excision and extension are performed according to the basic principles of hand surgery. A Lengemann suture is passed through the central stump of the extensor tendon slip, and the central stump is pulled distally until if joins with the peripheral stump. The wire is passed to the tip of the finger through a narrow channel drilled in the distal phalanx, where it is fastened over a small rubber disk. A sterile button serves best to prevent compressive damage to the soft tissue of the fingertip, as it distributes the pressure over a large area. Temporary drill-wire arthrodesis of the terminal joint for 5 weeks in hyperextension is recommended as a supplementary measure (Figure 83a,b).

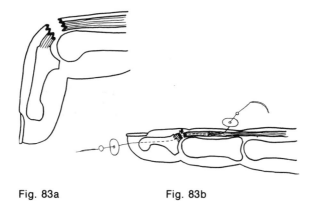

Fig. 83a   Fig. 83b

2. Open Injury of Extensor Tendon
   with Bone Involvement

The procedure is similar to that described above. The Lengemann suture is passed through or over the bone fragment. The wire is removed after 5 weeks (Figure 84a,b).

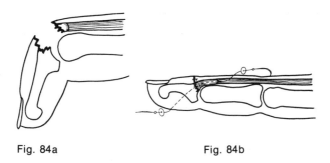

Fig. 84a   Fig. 84b

3. Fresh Closed Extensor Tendon Rupture
   without Bone Involvement

The opening of the rupture is about 5 mm wide when the basal and middle joints are extended. When the terminal joint is hyperextended and the middle joint is flexed, the opening shrinks to 1–2 mm. If the basal joint is also flexed, the proximal tendon stump overrides the distal stump by 2 mm. The conservative Mommsen treatment as modified by Wilhelm is based on these anatomical facts: A circular forearm cast with plaster palm piece on which the injured finger is immobilized with adhesive plaster strips is used for 5 weeks. The basal and middle joints are fixed in 90° flexion, and the terminal joint in hyperextension (Figure 85a,b).

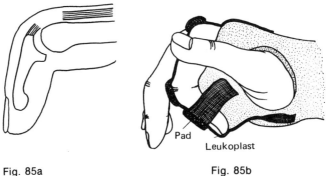

Fig. 85a   Fig. 85b

This arrangement is complicated, somewhat annoying and not at all as successful as is believed. Better results can be obtained with minimal discomfort by temporary drill-wire arthrodesis of the terminal joint in hyperextension and the middle joint in flexion, provided the injury is not old when treated: A drill wire 1 mm in diameter is drilled in longitudinally from the tip of the finger close to the nail, but without damaging the nail bed. To maintain the desired joint position through the drilling procedure, the surgeon holds the injured finger such that his ring finger rests on the dorsal side of the proximal phalanx, his middle finger is beneath the flexed middle joint, his index finger rests on the dorsal side of the terminal joint, and his thumb keeps the terminal joint in hyperextension by pressure on the bulb of the finger. An adjunctive Böhler splint protects the fingertip against inadvertant shock for 1 week. The wire is removed after 5 weeks (Figure 86).

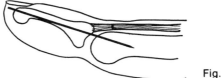

Fig. 86

4. Fresh Closed Extensor Tendon Rupture with Bone Involvement

This can also be treated exclusively by temporary drill-wire arthrodesis. Better, however, is the anatomically precise operative adaptation of the fragment from a right-angle incision by means of a Lengemann suture and temporary drill-wire arthrodesis (Figure 87a,b).

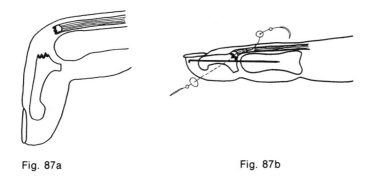

Fig. 87a   Fig. 87b

5. Old Extensor Slip Injuries

A rupture may be considered "old" after only 1 week if it is no longer amenable to conservative treatment or temporary drill-wire arthrodesis. In this case, shortening of the tendon slip which has been lengthened by scar tissue is the only recourse. The following technique is used:

a. Purse-String Suture after Georg
A right-angle incision is used. The scar length is shortened by mersilene 4/0 pulled in an elliptical path after mobilization of the undersurface. Temporary drill-wire arthrodesis of the terminal joint is removed after 5 weeks (Figure 88a,b).

b. Folding of the Extensor Tendon Slip
by the Pulvertaft Method
A right-angle incision is made over the middle phalanx. The intact region of the extensor slip is exposed and folded over with mersilene 5/0 such that it is sufficiently shortened. Temporary drill-wire arthrodesis of the terminal joint is removed after 5 weeks (Figure 89).

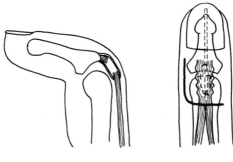

Fig. 88a   Fig. 88b

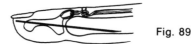

Fig. 89

Defect injuries call for the plastic operations of Iselin and Nichols. Arthrodesis of the terminal joint is safer in such cases (for technique see Section VIII,B,2,a).

VIII. Injury of the Deep Flexor Tendon in the Fingertip Region

A. Diagnosis

The terminal joint is extended and cannot be actively flexed. The closed bony avulsion of the deep flexor tendon from the distal phalanx may be caused by sudden hyperextension. More common is an open, sharp division distal to the passage of the deep flexor tendon through the superficial flexor tendon, which is to say at the level of the middle phalanx. While the bony avulsion is not especially prone to retraction, the central tendon stump resulting from a sharp division usually retracts a considerable distance palmarward. The bony avulsion requires immediate operative treatment. The divided deep tendon, on the other hand, must not be sutured in the interest of preserving the gliding ability of the superficial tendon. In these cases, arthrodesis (or tenodesis) of the terminal joint should be undertaken to stabilize this joint. An effort is made to fuse the joint in the position best suited to the individual occupational needs of the patient. This must be discussed with the patient beforehand! A tendon graft involving the sacrifice of the superficial flexor tendon is out of the question in view of the known problems associated with replacement of the flexor tendons.

B. Treatment

The technique for treating the bony avulsion of the deep tendon is basically as follows: The tendon fragment, which is under proximal tension, is fixed by means of strong pull-out wire in such a way that no retraction is possible even during exertion of the muscle or in the position of function.

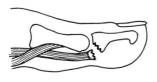

Fig. 90a

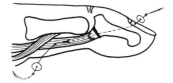

Fig. 90b

1. Bony Avulsion of the Deep Tendon

A midlateral longitudinal incision is always made on the ulnar side of the index and middle fingers. The tendon sheath is opened if necessary. A Lengemann suture is placed through the tendon near the bone fragment and passed through the fragment or beneath it; it then follows a channel drilled through the distal phalanx to its exit point distal to the lunula on the nail. After accurate reduction, the suture is tightly anchored over a button or rubber disk. The suture is removed after 3 weeks (Figure 90a,b).

2. Division of the Deep Tendon

a. Arthrodesis of the Terminal Joint

The terminal joint is opened by a transverse or right-angle incision on the dorsal side. The articular surfaces are resected by saw, taking into account the angle of fusion desired. The resection surfaces are approximated (with arthrodetic forceps, if available) and fixed with two short, parallel Kirschner wires 0.8–1 mm in diameter, which are drilled in longitudinally. The ends of the wires are snipped off below skin level and buried. A plaster splint applied on the dorsal side will protect the fingertip against inadvertant shocks for 8–10 days. The wires are removed after full union of the arthrodetic surfaces has occurred (Figure 91a,b).

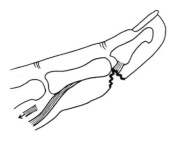

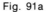

Fig. 91a

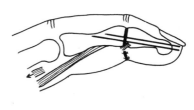

Fig. 91b

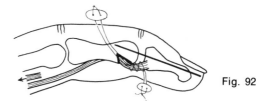

Fig. 92

b. Tenodesis of the Terminal Joint (Moberg)

A midlateral longitudinal incision opening the tendon sheath is made. The distal tendon stump is armed with a 4/0 multifilament pull-out wire. A notch is made with a chisel below the head of the middle phalanx. The tendon stump is pulled into the notch with the wire such that the desired position is obtained. The wire itself is passed through a bone channel to the dorsal side, where it is tied off over a button. The terminal joint is stabilized by temporary drill-wire arthrodesis (Figure 92). If the distal tendon stump is too short, of course, only arthrodesis remains.

IX. Traumatic Epithelial Cyst

This type of cyst tends to afflict the fingertip and amputation stumps, and occurs more rarely in the palm. It appears as a tender, subcutaneous nodule and is formed by the traumatic displacement of proliferative epithelial tissue, usually as the result of fine puncture wounds, which may be quite old. In rare cases it may reach the size of a cherry, erode the bone, and lead to spontaneous fracture, thereby raising the suspicion of a true neoplasm. These cysts interfere with grasp and require operative removal. Bony defects are filled with autologous cancellous grafts from the iliac crest.

Bibliography

Atasoy, E., et al.: Reconstruction of the amputated finger tip with a tringular volar flap. J. Bone Joint Surg. A 52, 921 (1970).

Brody, G. S., Cloutier, A. M., Woolhouse, F. M.: The finger tip injury and assessment of management. Plast. Reconstr. Surg. 26, 80 (1960).

Frank, E.: Ergebnisse der konservativen Behandlung der subcutanen Strecksehnen ausrisse an den Fingern. Chir. Praxis 1, 531 (1957).

Georg, H.: Zur Behandlung der geschlossenen Strecksehnenabrisse am Fingerendglied. Langenbecks Arch. Chir. 292, 485 (1959).

Horner, R. L.: Finger tip trauma. Surg. Clin. North Am. 49, 1373 (1969).

Kruhl, E., Stimming, W.: Typische Fingerverletzungen beim Ballspielen. Monatsschr. Unfallheilkd. 67, 478 (1964).

Mittelbach, H. R.: Fingerendgliedverletzungen. Chirurg 37, 306 (1966).

Mommsen, R.: Muskelphysiologie der Fingerstrecker und Verbandbehandlung des Strecksehnenabrisses am Endgelenk. Zentralbl. Chir. 79, 265 (1954).

Neumann, H.: Zur Verletzung des Fingerendgliedes und dessen biologische Shienung durch Nagelplastik. Monatsschr. Unfallheilkd. 66, 398 (1963).

Pratt, D. R.: Internal splint for closed and open treatment of injuries of extensor tendons at distal joint of fingers. J. Bone Joint Surg. A 34, 785 (1952).

Recht, P.: Ästhetische Gesichtspunkte der Chirurgie der Fingerendglieder. Langenbecks Arch. Chir. 299, 105 (1961).

Snow, J. W.: Isolated fingertip injuries. J. Fla. Med. Assoc. 55, 820 (1968).

Walcher, K.: Zum subcutanen Riß der Streckaponeurose über dem Endgelenk der Langfinger und des Daumens. Chirurg 39, 431 (1968).

Soft Tissue Injuries of the Dorsal Side

Injuries of the Wrist Extensors, Long Finger Extensor Tendons, and Dorsal Aponeurosis of the Fingers

The progress made in the area of flexor tendon surgery of the hand since Bunnell has unjustly placed the extensor tendons somewhat in the background due to their relatively simple sheath structures. Functional losses due to extensor tendon injuries may not be as serious in general as flexor lesions, but the proper interaction between flexors and extensors is essential for differentiated grasp. The suture or transfer of an extensor tendon on the back of the hand or in the carpal region presents few difficulties, especially when the suture techniques proved in flexor tendon surgery are applied to the extensors. Here the functional losses are minimal, however, owing to the presence of tendinous junctions (Figure 93). Only distal to the tendinous junctions are real difficulties encountered. Knowledge gained during the past decade on the anatomy and the physiological as well as pathological motor characteristics of the extensor apparatus of the fingers has again placed the surgical importance of this system in its proper light.

In preparing the operating plan for the care of fresh or long-standing extensor tendon injuries, the surgeon must realize that extension of the long fingers, and thus the opening of the hand, plays a secondary role to flexion during grasping; the importance of this role varies with the occupation of the patient. Thus, partial extension is one or sometimes two finger joints may be acceptable in some cases if the adjacent joints are able to compensate. It should be remembered that the post-traumatic flexion of a middle joint is relatively quickly compensated for by hyperextensibility of the basal joint, even in older persons. The stability of the grip and freedom from pain are of the highest priority, however. The primary operative stiffening of a joint whose natural functions can-

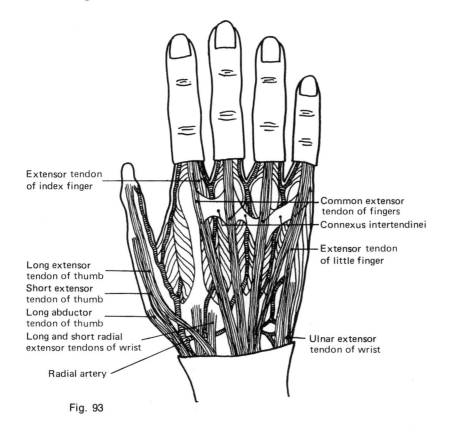

Extensor tendon
of index finger

Common extensor
tendon of fingers

Connexus intertendinei

Extensor tendon
of little finger

Long extensor
tendon of thumb

Short extensor
tendon of thumb

Long abductor
tendon of thumb

Long and short radial
extensor tendons of wrist

Ulnar extensor
tendon of wrist

Radial artery

Fig. 93

not be restored often makes it possible to preserve a useful finger, sometimes shortens the treatment time considerably, and prevents the damage that would result from spontaneous stiffening in an unfavorable
position or amputation. An analysis of the occupational needs of the patient is essential. No single rule can be given for the "most favorable"
position, but it generally ranges from 130° to 150°.

Before going into technical details, we must discuss a few basics:

1)   In smooth divisions of skin and tendon in one plane and in areas
not subjected to strong tension (i.e., in the region of the proximal and
middle phalanx), the skin and tendon can be sutured concurrently by
several figure-of-eight sutures (Figure 94). Otherwise the transversely
severed tendon is treated according to the "suture at a distance" principle with a Lengemann suture (Figure 95a). The routine use of the Len-
gemann-type suture at a distance to relieve tension on the tendon suture
permits the member to be immobilized in the position of function,
thereby shortening postoperative care and preventing joint stiffness.

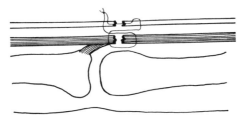

Fig. 94

The wire is removed by first disinfecting its distal end and clipping it off below the button. Then the central end of the wire is grasped with a clamp, and the wire is withdrawn with a quick pull (Figure 95b). Extensor tendons that are split longitudinally by accident or operative necessity are united by a continuous suture whose ends are passed through the skin and anchored over a button (Figure 96). Proximal to the wrist, a buried suture (Dychno-Bunnell) with 4/0 multifilament steel wire is indicated (Figure 97). Postoperative immobilization is maintained for 3 weeks.

2)   The operating field must be clearly visible in extensor tendon surgery. Extensions of fresh wounds and adequate access in reconstructive operations are therefore essential. These procedures must naturally follow the principles laid down by Bunnell in order to avoid dermatogenic contractures. Care must be taken to preserve all portions of the superficial branch of the radial nerve because they may be of great functional importance with regard to surgical reconstruction of the thumb.

3)   A good, scar-free skin covering is essential if the tendons are to glide properly. This is particularly true for the dorsal side of the hand

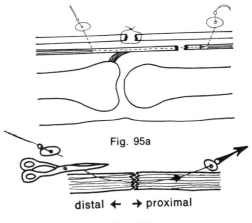

Fig. 95a

distal ← → proximal

Fig. 95b

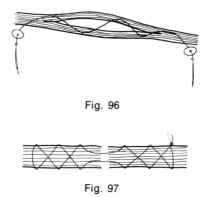

Fig. 96

Fig. 97

and fingers. Contracted scars that adhere to the tendons jeopardize the success of tendon repair. Moreover, poor scars on the dorsal side of the hand often result in painful cicatricial keloids. Skin grafting must therefore always be considered when the operating plan is formed.

4)   Accompanying bone injuries must be corrected by osteosynthesis in order to avoid malunions that impair muscle balance and to permit prompt therapeutic exercise.

I. Wrist Extensors

There are no motor losses and diagnosis is based on inspection of the wound. Isolated injuries are relatively rare. The loss of only one wrist extensor has at most a weakening effect, since stabilization of the wrist is ensured by the remaining extensor tendons. Nevertheless, a suture is indicated, especially in the case of the manual laborer. The central tendon stumps retract and must be located by means of an auxiliary incision. If the injury is near the insertion, the tendon is united by Lengemann suture (Figure 95); otherwise the Dychno-Bunnell technique with 4/0 multifilament steel wire is employed (Figure 97). The wrist is immobilized in the position of function for 3 weeks.

II. Division of the Long Finger Extensors Central
to the Tendinous Junctions

If only one tendon is injured, there is at most a slight loss of extension in the basal joint. This loss increases if several tendons are injured simultaneously.

The extensor tendons usually retract little in the region of the dorsum, but tend to retract considerably in the region of the wrist and distal forearm. The central tendon stumps are therefore located by means of auxiliary incisions. Blind "fishing" for tendon stumps is to be avoided.

Union in the region of the dorsum is accomplished by Lengemann suture, with 3/0 atraumatic Dexon sutures used for fine adaptation of the stumps. The corresponding tendon compartment in the region of the dorsal carpal ligament is split in order to prevent adhesions. In the forearm, buried 4/0 multifilament steel wire sutures are applied by the Dychno-Bunnell method. The wrist and long fingers are immobolized in the position of function for 3 weeks.

III. Division of the Extensor Tendons in the Region of the Metacarpophalangeal Joint

The finger cannot be actively extended in the metacarpophalangeal joint.

Treatment is by a stress-relieving "suture at a distance" with a Lengemann suture, with 3/0 atraumatic Dexon sutures used for fine adaptation. If the cutaneous wound and tendon division lie in the same plane, the tendon stumps can be adapted and the skin simultaneously closed by figure-of-eight sutures with mersilene 4/0. Here, too, the extremity is immobilized for 3 weeks in the position of function. The stitches are pulled after the cast is removed.

Not every loss of extension in the metacarpophalangeal joint is the result of a direct tendon injury. Dislocation of the extensor tendon associated with a closed rupture or open division of the interosseous hood may create the same picture. In this case the dorsal side of the metacarpophalangeal joint must be broadly exposed to provide an adequate view of the complex anatomy of the extensor apparatus. The divisions are repaired with 3/0 atraumatic Dexon sutures, a procedure which is successful even for long-standing injuries. This procedure is followed by immobilization in plaster for 3 weeks in the position of function.

IV. Division of the Dorsal Aponeurosis in the Region of the Proximal and Middle Phalanges

Two motor systems are active in this region: the long extensors and the system of intrinsic hand muscles that act on the three finger joints.

The tendons of the common extensor muscle, interosseous muscles, and lumbrical muscles, joined together by ligaments and fibrous plates, form the dorsal aponeurosis, which extends the middle joint with an intermediate tract inserted into the base of the middle phalanx, and the distal joint with the lateral slips that converge at the terminal joint. Landsmeer's ligaments, which radiate obliquely from the flexor tendon sheath at the level of the proximal phalanx to the lateral tracts at the level of the middle joint and middle phalanx, are of particular importance for the mechanics of the two interphalangeal joints. The ligament transmits the force of one extensor and one flexor to these joints with its dynamic tenodesis effect (Wilhelm; Figure 98a,b).

A fresh injury to these delicate structures, whether it involves a closed rupture or an open division unaccompanied by defect formation, presents no particular operative difficulties. However, adequate exposure of the injured area is necessary if anatomical reconstruction is to be performed.

Particular attention should be given divisions of the intermediate tract at the middle joint in order to prevent the *boutonnière deformity*—a condition in which the lateral slips of the extensor apparatus are displaced below the plane of the middle joint and thus act as flexors of this joint, while simultaneously hyperextending the terminal joint.

During treatment, the middle slip is kept from retracting by Lengemann suture, while button sutures of 3/0 atraumatic Dexon are used for fine adaptation of the other structures. Figure-of-eight sutures have

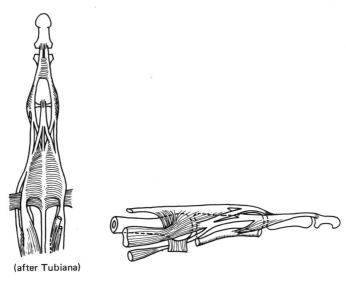

(after Tubiana)

Fig. 98a   Fig. 98b

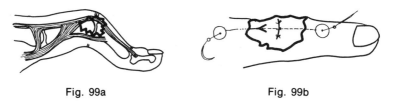

Fig. 99a   Fig. 99b

proved useful if the skin wound and tendon suture are in the same plane. The suture leads to a slight flexion in the basal joint, while the interphalangeal joints are extended. The fingers are also splinted in this position for 5 weeks (Figure 99a,b). Distal to the middle joint, the extensor aponeurosis is joined with figure-of-eight sutures.

There is ample documentation to show that long-standing injuries and fresh defect injuries in the region of the middle joint are problematic from a surgical standpoint. Wilhelm's procedure for long-standing injuries is attractive due to its simplicity, but it is applicable only if no tissue defects are present. The dorsal side of the middle joint is exposed by a lateral curved longitudinal incision. The tendon stumps are avived. The pull of the intermediate tract is eliminated by Lengemann suture. Individual button sutures with Dexon 3/0 are used for fine adaptation. The basal joint is splinted in slight flexion and the interphalangeal joints in extension for 5 weeks (Figure 100).

A brilliant technique is that of Littler and Eaton, whereby the entire extensile force of the extensors and interossei is transmitted to the base of the middle phalanx, and the rest of the aponeurotic segment that extends the terminal joint is relaxed by leaving extension of the terminal joint to Landsmeer's ligaments and, on the radial side, to the lumbrical muscle. This procedure is also suitable for correcting minor defects and is successful even when skin conditions are poor. Broad exposure of the extensor aponeurosis is accomplished by an S-shaped longitudinal incision. The segments of the dorsal aponeurosis arising from the extensor slips and the interosseous muscles are completely separated from Landsmeer's ligaments and the lumbrical nerve. With the middle joint in full extension, the sides are folded inward and joined together by loop sutures of Dexon 3/0. If necessary, they are also sutured to the base of the middle phalanx. The middle joint is stabilized in extension for 2 weeks

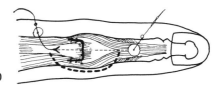

Fig. 100

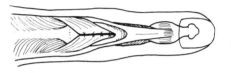

Fig. 101

by temporary drill-wire arthrodesis. The finger is immobilized for 1 additional week (Figure 101).

Larger defects call for techniques that make use of free-grafted tendon slips. The classic Fowler graft can still be used in such cases. It is certainly better than its reputation, although good skin conditions are requisite for its use. These can, if necessary, be created by preliminary plastic measures. This technique involves removal of a palmar tendon. Bilateral longitudinal incisions are made in the central third of the middle phalanx and bilateral angular incisions in the central half of the proximal phalanx. From here the surgeon tunnels under the dorsal side of the middle joint. Centrally, the tendons of the interosseous muscles are exposed on both sides, and distally the lateral slips of the extensor aponeurosis are exposed. The latter are lifted from their bed for a small portion of their length. The palmar tendon is pulled through this tunnel, crossed beneath the skin at the level of the middle joint, passed through the tunnel of skin, and quilt-stitched to the interosseous tendons on both sides with Dexon 3/0 loop sutures. The finger is immobilized for 5 weeks in a cast with the basal joint in slight flexion and the interphalangeal joints in a extension (Figure 102).

V. Extensor Tendon Injuries with Accompanying Bone Injuries

Such injuries are sometimes seen in sawing accidents and severe crush injuries inflicted by machinery. For the tendon suture to be successful, the muscle balance must not be impaired by skeletal malunions. Accompanying bone injuries must therefore be treated by osteosynthesis (see the chapter on Fractures).

If the articular surfaces of the middle and basal joints are destroyed, two treatment techniques are available: arthrodesis and arthroplasty.

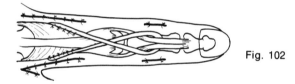

Fig. 102

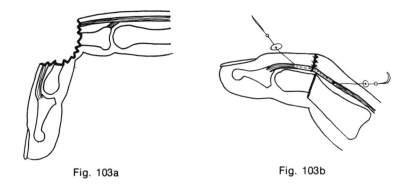

Fig. 103a   Fig. 103b

Arthrodesis is preferred for the middle joint, while arthroplasty can be attempted on the basal joint before other measures are taken. At present, we are still somewhat skeptical of efforts to permanently restore the mobility of injured joints by alloarthroplastic means. Certainly this technique is as little suited for daily practice as the autoplastic transfer of toe joints or joints from amputated fingers. Whatever approach is taken, however, an attempt should be made to restore the tendons so that at least the remaining joints will have a certain degree of mobility. Arthrodesis is performed according to the rules previously discussed for the terminal joint (Figure 103a,b). It should be pointed out that arthrodesis of the middle and terminal joints is sometimes the only means of preserving a useful, although shortened, finger provided there is sufficient mobility in the basal joint. This is especially true for the index finger.

Arthroplasty (Figures 143, 144) will be discussed in more detail in the chapter on Fractures.

Bibliography

Dolphin, J. A.: The extensor tenotomy for chronic boutonnière deformity of the finger. J. Bone Joint Surg. A 47, 161 (1965).
Fowler, S. B.: The management of tendon injuries. J. Bone Joint Surg. A 41, 579 (1959).
Gülgönen, A., Vlasich, E.: Strecksehnendurchtrennungen der Hand. Chir. Praxis 13, 111 (1969).
Hellman, K.: Die Wiederherstellung der Strecksehnen im Bereich der Fingermittelgelenke. Langenbecks Arch. Chir. 309, 36 (1965).
Kettelkamp, D. J., Flatt, K. E., Moulds, R.: Traumatic dislocations of the long-finger extensor tendon. J. Bone Joint Surg. A. 53, 229 (1971).
Landsmeer, J. M. F.: The anatomy of the dorsal aponeurosis of the human finger and its functional significance. Anat. Rec. 104, 31 (1943).
Littler, J. W.: The finger extensor mechanism. Surg. Clin. North Am. 47, 415 (1967).

Littler, J. W., Cooley, S. G. E.: Restoration of the retinacular system in hyperextension deformity of the proximal interphalangeal joint. J. Bone Joint Surg. A 47, 637 (1965).

Littler, J. W., Eaton, R. G.: Redistribution of forces in the correction of the boutonnière deformity. J. Bone Joint Surg. A 49, 1267 (1967).

Matev, J.: Transposition of the lateral slips of the aponeurosis in treatment of the long-standing "boutonnieère deformity" of the fingers. Br. J. Plast. Surg. 17, 281 (1964).

Michow, J., Vichsed, P.: Luxations latérales des tendons extenseur en regard de l'articulation métacarpophalangienne. Rev. Méd. Nancy 86, 595 (1961).

Mittelbach, H. R.: Strecksehnenverletzungen an der Hand. Bericht über die Behandlung von 159 Fällen. Chirurg 34, 169 (1963).

Tubiana, R.: Surgical repair of the extensor apparatus of the fingers. Surg. Clin. North Am. 48, 1050 (1968).

Tubiana, R., Valentin, P.: The anatomy of the extensor apparatus of the fingers. Surg. Clin. North Am. 44, 897 (1964).

Tubiana, R., Valentin, P.: The physiology of the extensor apparatus of the fingers. Surg. Clin. North Am. 44, 907 (1964).

Wheeldon, F. Z.: Recurrent dislocation of extensor tendons in the hand. J. Bone Joint Surg. B 36, 612 (1954).

Wilhelm, A.: Neue Operationstechniken in der Strecksehnenchirurgie. Chir. Plast. Reconstr. 6, 23 (1969).

Soft Tissue Injuries of the Volar Side

Injuries of the Long Finger Flexor Tendons, Wrist Flexors, and Median and Ulnar Nerves

The prognosis of these injuries depends basically on whether and to what extent the functionally critical anatomical structures of this region (flexor tendons and nerves) have been damaged (Figure 104). Every wound on the volar side of the hand raises the possibility of an accompanying tendon or nerve injury, and the division need not lie in the plane of the skin injury. Glass splinter wounds are particularly notorious in this regard.

The diagnosis of a fresh flexor tendon or nerve division must be made by careful examination *before* care is administered so that the operation can be properly planned.

I. Flexor Tendon Surgery

1) Reconstructive surgery following flexor tendon injuries can be problematic, especially in the region of the tendon sheaths ("no man's land"; Figure 105), because for a sutured area to heal or a tendon graft to take, vascularized connective tissue must approach the tendon from its surroundings. This leads to fibrous growths between the tendon surface and its sheath, ranging from delicate, innocuous adhesions to massive scars that can permanently prevent the tendon from gliding.

2) The extent of scar formation and thus the result of treatment is dependent on the following:

a) The nature and localization of the injury and the individual tendency to cicatrization.

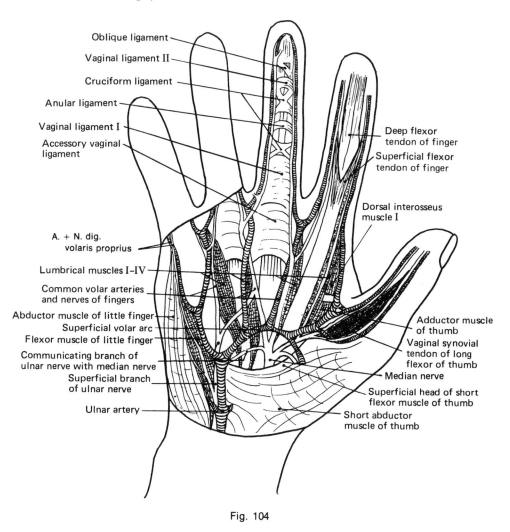

Oblique ligament
Vaginal ligament II
Cruciform ligament
Anular ligament
Vaginal ligament I
Accessory vaginal ligament

Deep flexor tendon of finger
Superficial flexor tendon of finger

Dorsal interosseus muscle I

A. + N. dig. volaris proprius
Lumbrical muscles I–IV
Common volar arteries and nerves of fingers
Abductor muscle of little finger
Superficial volar arc
Flexor muscle of little finger
Communicating branch of ulnar nerve with median nerve
Superficial branch of ulnar nerve
Ulnar artery

Adductor muscle of thumb
Vaginal synovial tendon of long flexor of thumb
Median nerve
Superficial head of short flexor muscle of thumb
Short abductor muscle of thumb

Fig. 104

b)   The technique of operative care.

Thus, smooth incised wounds have a better prognosis than severe mangling injuries. A traumatizing operative technique and improper procedures also worsen the prognosis. The following factors are therefore especially important for successful flexor tendon surgery:

a)   Appropriate measures are taken to relieve pain.
b)   Adequate access is attained to the rules of hand surgery. It should

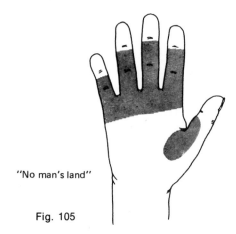

"No man's land"

Fig. 105

be remembered that the central tendon stumps may retract considerably. They must be located by auxiliary incision.
c) A clearly visible and thus bloodless operating field must be ensured;
    otherwise, tendon and nerve stumps may be inadvertently joined to-
    gether.
d) An atraumatic technique is used employing extremely fine instru-
    ments.
e) The tissue is kept moist by irrigation with Ringer's solution.
f) The tendon sheaths are not touched, if possible.
g) The tendon surface should not be touched. A graft may be handled
    only by its ends. Areas that are unavoidably traumatized are excised
    after anastomosis of the tendon.
h) Only sparing use of moist swabs is permissible.

   3) The suture material lays a special role in flexor tendon surgery:

a) It must be compatible with the tissue as well as nonabsorbable and
    must not swell. Plastic filament and stainless steel wire are accept-
    able.
b) It must be as fine as possible and possess adequate tensile strength.
    Suture sizes 4/0 or 5/0 are correct, depending on the tendon dimen-
    sions.

   4) The suturing technique must be appropriate for the tissue conditions:

a) Distal attachment of a graft is performed with transosseal pull-out
    wire by Bunnell's method (Figure 106a–d).

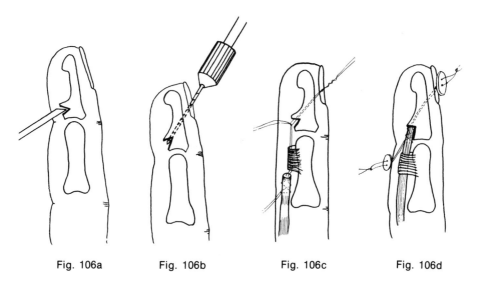

Fig. 106a   Fig. 106b   Fig. 106c   Fig. 106d

b)   Union of the thinner central graft stump with the thicker central flexor tendon stump is accomplished by Pulvertaft's technique of interweaving (Figure 107a–e).

c)   If both tendon ends have the same cross section, they can be joined end-to-end by the Dychno-Bunnell bootlace technique (Figure 108a,b).

d)   For primary suture in "no man's land," the "suture at a distance"

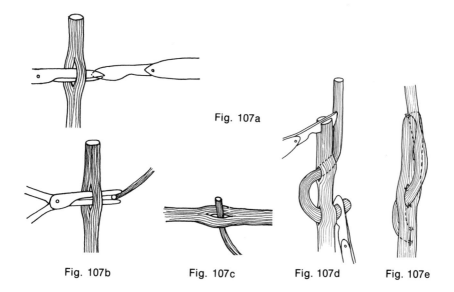

Fig. 107a

Fig. 107b   Fig. 107c   Fig. 107d   Fig. 107e

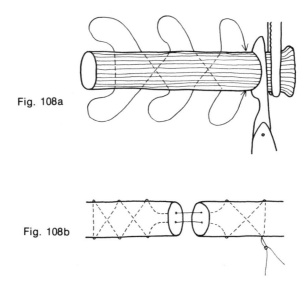

Fig. 108a

Fig. 108b

(Lengemann, Bunnell) or Bsteh's blocking technique (Figures 109–111) is recommended to relieve stress on the central tendon stump. The suture area is then adapted with two fine Dexon 3/0 sutures.

5)   The tendon surface and tendon graft need time and rest to heal. Absolute immobilization for at least 3 weeks in plaster in the position of function ensures undisturbed tendon healing and prevents unnecessary scar formation and contractures.
6)   Divided superficial flexor tendons should not be sutured.
7)   Partial divisions require no suture.

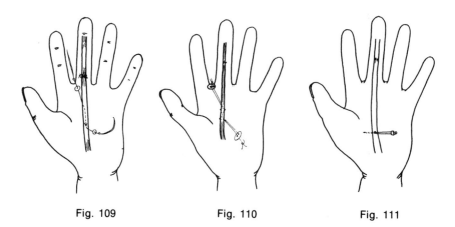

Fig. 109   Fig. 110   Fig. 111

8)   Aftercare is as important as operative care. It requires empathy, persistence, and patience on the part of the physician, and the will to recover, intelligence, and patience on the part of the patient. Active equipment-assisted exercise under the supervision of a physical therapist is of paramount importance. Operative tendolysis may improve a poor result in some cases.

9)   No one is immune to poor results in flexor tendon surgery. It should be remembered, however, that a long finger that is stiffened in the position of function and has sensation is by no means useless as long as the mobility of the basal joint, which of course is independent of flexor tendon function, can be preserved; otherwise an amputation in the interest of overall hand function cannot be avoided.

II. Neurosurgery

1)   Only rarely can the stumps of a severed nerve be adapted so precisely by the conventional epineural suture (Figure 112) that adaptation of the fascicles is also achieved and normal axon regeneration can occur.

2)   The formation of fibrous connections between the nerve stumps due to inadequate resection of the damaged nerve segments also hinders axon regeneration.

3)   Tension in the suture area leads to cicatrization and also impedes regeneration. A "tension-free" suture achieved by immobilizing the joints in an extreme stress-relieved position only postpones the problem of nerve stretch injuries until the joints are released.

4)   Microsurgical techniques (fascicular suture; Figure 113) employing autologous nerve grafts have greatly improved the prognosis of nerve divisions in recent times. The sheathing of nerve suture (Millipore), on the other hand, has produced disappointing results.

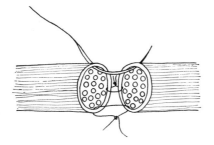

Fig. 112

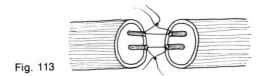

Fig. 113

III. Position of the Beginner, the Experienced Surgeon, and the Specialist in the Treatment of Flexor Tendon and Nerve Injuries of the Hand

As in operative treatment of fractures, there is both an objective and subjective indication for reconstructive measures. The former pertains to the local facilities available and the nature of the injury, and the latter to the surgeon himself. Only if both indications are present there is a reasonable prospect of success. The physician requires both insight and self-criticism to make such a judgment.

A. Beginner

The novice must limit himself to primary wound closure, including the care of accompanying bone injuries if necessary. If this overtaxes his abilities in complicated cases, he will in no way incur the disrespect of reasonable colleagues by asking a more experienced surgeon for help and advice. The faulty evaluation of the situation and one's own abilities may have regrettable consequences for the patient.

B. Experienced Surgeon

There is no reason why the "accomplished" surgeon should not perform all routine operations on the flexor tendons, including primary suture, provided his knowledge of the techniques and methods of hand surgery is derived from experience and he is willing to spend the time required for such operations, which may be quite lengthy.

C. Hand Specialist

Regrafting of the flexor tendons, grafting after tendon necrosis, tendolysis, and reconstructive microsurgery on the nerves are procedures best left to the specialist.

IV. Treatment Tactics for Routine Practice

1) Tension-free wound closure and primary wound healing with the avoidance of dermatogenic contractures are essential for the success of operations on the flexor tendons and nerves. They may require primary plastic measures.

2) Accompanying bone injuries require osteosynthesis before the flexor tendons and nerves are treated.

3) Opened tendon sheaths are left alone.

4) Secondary, possibly bilateral flexor tendon grafting is the procedure of choice. It can generally be performed 4–8 weeks after the injury, assuming primary healing of the wound, but may be successfully undertaken later as long as the unavoidable atrophy of the motor muscle has not progressed too far. After 1 year, grafting becomes problematic.

5) In the case of smooth incised wounds, primary suture of the deep tendon may be undertaken in "no man's land," but only by the experienced surgeon.

6) Primary suture of the deep tendon is contraindicated for severe mangling injuries of the soft parts of the hand and is problematic in the wrist area.

7) The careful primary epineural adaptation of the nerve stumps is permitted. Even a successful neurosuture can be achieved by this procedure in some cases. In any event, anatomical orientation during the reconstructive operation is facilitated.

8) Microsurgery on the severed nerve is indicated if it is found that the adjacent nerves cannot compensate for the functional loss, and this loss is severe.

9) Motor and sensory transfers after nerve injuries are still justifiable even in the age of microsurgery.

V. Operative Techniques

A. Injury in "No Man's Land" on the Volar Side of a Long Finger

If active flexion of the middle and terminal joints is impossible but the basal joint can still be actively moved, a division of both flexor tendons is present. If only the terminal joint cannot be actively flexed, the deep tendon alone is severed. Slight wiggling movements triggered by cords of connective tissue may create the impression of intact tendons. An isolated superficial tendon injury has a weakening effect but causes no direct functional loss. The tendon injury is frequently accompanied by damage to the volar neurovascular bundles. It should be noted that *one* intact volar artery is sufficient to ensure nutrition of the finger.

1. Division of Both Flexor Tendons with
   Replacement of the Profundus Tendon by a Free Graft
   (Palmaris Tendon, Toe Extensor, Plantaris Tendon)
   in One Operation

1)   The time to operate has come when the finger joints can be freely moved passively and nonirritating scar conditions are present. This situation exists after 3–4 weeks at the earliest.

2)   Exposure is by midlateral longitudinal incision on the dorsal side of the neurovascular bundle, with an auxiliary incision in the palm or exposure by Bruner's method (Figure 114).

3)   The tendon sheath is excised while the annular ligaments are preserved.

4)   The distal tendon stumps are removed.

5)   The graft is taken; complete exposure is the most atraumatic method.

6)   The graft is drawn into place.

7)   Length determination and fixation are performed. The graft must span at least the distance from the terminal joint to the palm beyond the central boundary of "no man's land." The length is determined by fixing the graft on the distal phalanx with transosseal pull-out wire (Figure 106) and joining it with the central profundus stump by the method of Pulvertaft (Figure 107) in such a way that the finger assumes a correct resting position relative to the adjacent fingers. For several years we have preferred the technique of Rank and Wakefield as modi-

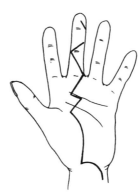

Fig. 114

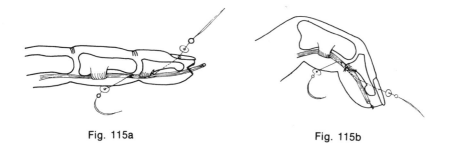

Fig. 115a   Fig. 115b

fied by Stenström, whereby the central anastomosis is applied first (Figure 115a,b).

8) The tourniquet is loosened before closure of the wound, and suturing is deferred until reactive hyperemia has subsided. Complete removal of the cuff prevents hyperemic bleeding. As a rule, no significant bleeding occurs if the incisions are correctly placed. If it becomes necessary to arrest the bleeding, this is done by point microcoagulation. Ligatures should not be employed. Secretions are drained for 24 hours by a Redon drain inserted into the wound area. This drain must not touch the tendon.

9) The wound is sutured only by button suture of the skin. These sutures are tied only tight enough to evenly appose the wound edges and must remain loose enough not to cut into the skin when postoperative edema develops.

10) Postoperatively, the part is immobilized in the position of function by means of a dorsal plaster splint, with the wrist in the stress-relieved position. The arm is elevated after the operation. The cast and pull-out wire are removed after 3 weeks. This is followed by exercise.

2. Division of Both Flexor Tendons with Replacement of the Profundus Tendon in Two Operations

This technique has significantly improved the prognosis of flexor tendon grafts.

1) In the first session, the graft bed is prepared as in single-stage grafting. Instead of a tendon graft, a Silastic tube is inserted, about which a sheath will form in 8–10 weeks.

2) In the second session, the implant is removed and replaced with the tendon graft by the usual technique. This step requires only that the beginning and end of the newly formed sheath be exposed.

3. Division of Both Flexor Tendons with Primary Suture of the Profundus Tendon

Primary suture of the profundus in "no man's land" is possible for the experienced surgeon. We agree with Buck-Gramcko, however, that "no man's land" should by no means become "every man's land."

1) The area of the injury is exposed.

2) The distal superficial tendon stump is removed.

3) The central stump of the deep tendon is located by auxiliary incision.

4) The deep tendon stumps are united after avivement with a razor blade by the "suture at a distance" technique or by blocking of the central tendon stump (Figures 109–111).

4. Isolated Division of the Deep Tendon

Primary suture or secondary grafting should be avoided in the interest of preserving the function of the superficial tendon (see chapter on Fingertip Injuries).

5. Isolated Division of the Superficial Tendon

Reunion is unnecessary. If cicatricial blockage of the deep tendon by the superficial tendon occurs during healing, the latter is surgically removed.

6. Division of a Neurovascular Bundle

Hemorrhages generally stop by themselves, rendering care of the vascular stumps unnecessary. In rare cases the vessels may be ligated with catgut 6/0, but point electrocoagulation of the vascular lumen is better. In cases of severed digital nerves, an attempt is made to restore continuity up to the level of the middle phalanx by primary epineural end-to-end suture after the nerve is avived by razor blade.

B. Injury in the Palm Outside "No Man's Land," in the Thenar or Hypothenar Region

The volar aponeurosis must not be sutured. Partial extirpation, as in the case of Dupuytren's contracture, is sometimes indicated.

Concomitant muscular injuries are common. Muscle tissue may not be sutured, but the delicate fasciae may be adapted if need be. Muscular sutures lead only to the destruction of more muscle tissues by ischemia.

1. Injuries of the Flexor Tendons

The same principles apply here as in injuries in "no man's land." The indications for primary suture of the deep tendon are somewhat broader than in "no man's land," however. As a rule, the superficial tendon is not sutured.

2. Vascular Injuries

Bleeding from the palmar arches requires 5/0 ligature of the vessels after the arterial stumps are cleanly exposed. This has no adverse effects on hand circulation.

3. Nerve Injuries

In addition to lesions of the sensory branches of the median and ulnar nerves, the possibility of damage to their motor branches must be taken into consideration and tested for. Division of the trunk of the ulnar nerve in the hypothenar region is not uncommon. The possibly undamaged motor branch of the median nerve is particularly susceptible to injury during the surgical treatment of palm injuries.

The nerve stumps may be adapted by epineural suture. Microsurgery and possibly transfer operations must also be included in the list of therapeutic considerations.

The extent of a hemorrhage or a nerve injury near the wrist may necessitate splitting the roof of the carpal tunnel or Guyon's canal in order to prevent compressive neuropathy.

C. Injury in the Carpal Region

Combined injuries are common. The surgeon must have a steady operating field and clear visibility. General or plexus anesthesia and a bloodless field are therefore essential.

The following structures might be divided:

1) The tendon of the long flexor muscle of the thumb (see the chapter on Thumb Injuries).
2) The tendon of the long palmar muscle.
3) The tendons of the radial and ulnar flexor muscles of the wrist.
4) The superficial flexor tendons of the fingers, arranged in two pairs with flexors two and five situated below flexors three and four (Figures 116, 117).
5) The deep flexor tendons of the fingers (these lie in a row at the base of the carpal canal below superficial flexors two and five).

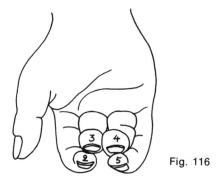

Fig. 116

6) The median and ulnar nerves.
7) The radial and ulnar arteries (Figure 117).

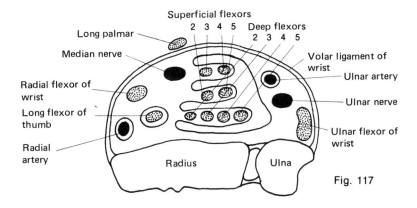

Fig. 117

1. Tendons

Primary care is desirable. The central stumps often retract far back into the hand. Broad exposure is required for localization and positive identification. Only in this way can the tissues be preserved and unfortunate anastomoses between nerve and tendon avoided.

Tendons not sutured are:

Long palmar.
Superficial flexor of the fingers.

Tendons that it is desirable but not absolutely necessary to suture are:

Radial flexor of the wrist.
Ulnar flexor of the wrist.

> **The continuity of the deep flexor tendon of the fingers and the long flexor tendon of the thumb must be restored.**

The suture is accomplished by end-to-end anastomosis by the bootlace technique of Dychno-Bunnell. This must be followed by immobilization in plaster with the fingers in the position of function and the wrist in the stress-relieved position for a period of 3 weeks.

Occasionally the peripheral stumps of the superficial flexor tendons will impede the gliding ability of the deep flexor tendons. They are therefore shortened initially so that they no longer lie in the scar region. They can always be removed during the second session if necessary.

2. Nerves

Like the tendons, the central nerve stumps retract and must be located by extension of the wound. The primary epineural suture is only rarely successful. Nevertheless, we favor it as a means of facilitating nerve location during the second operation, which can be performed after about 3 weeks if scar conditions are favorable. This is the domain of the early secondary suture of the fascicles, done with the aid of the operating microscope, or the nerve graft. Both are best left to the specialist.

If repair of the nerves is delayed for some reason, physiotherapeutic measures should be employed to prevent joint stiffening, and electrotherapy to ensure that the small muscles of the hand are kept in a functional state. *The suture of a motor nerve is doomed to failure if the organs served by it are no longer functional!*

3. Vessels

If only one of the two large arteries is severed, it can be ligated, since nutrition of the hand is ensured by the palmar arch. Division of both arteries does not necessarily seal the fate of the hand, but will definitely lead to a deficient blood supply. A vascular suture is indicated, therefore, even if it is problematic due to the relatively small vascular diameter. It should be attempted as soon as possible by an experienced surgeon, if available. It is unwise in such cases to proceed according to the principles of delayed primary care. Venous return is always ensured via the dorsum of the hand.

Bibliography

Anzel, S. H., Lipscomb, P. R., Grindlay, J. H.: Construction of artificial tendon sheaths in dogs. Am. J. Surg. 101, 355 (1961).

Arkin, A. M., Sieffert, R. S.: The use of wire in tenoplasty and tenorrhaphy. Am. J. Surg. 85, 795 (1953).

Biesalski, K.: Über Sehnenscheidenauswechslung. Dtsch. Med. Wochenschr. 36, 1615 (1910).

Boyes, J. H.: Immediate vs. delayed repair of the digital flexor tendons. Ann. West. Med. Surg. 1, 147 (1947).

Boyes, J. H.: Repair of the motor branch of the ulnar nerve in the palm. J. Bone Joint Surg. A 37, 920 (1955).

Brand, P. W.: Tendon grafting. J. Bone Joint Surg. B 43, 444 (1961).

Broder, H.: Rupture of flexor tendons associated with malunited Colles fracture. J. Bone Joint Surg. A 37, 404 (1955).

Brown, P. W.: Lacerations of the flexor tendons of the hand. Surg. Clin. North Am. 49, 1255 (1969).

Bsteh, O.: Sehnentransfixation bei Sehnendurchtrennungen. Chir. Praxis 2, 317 (1958).

Buck-Grmacko, D.: Probleme der Behandlung der Beugesehnenverletzungen. Chir. Praxis 11, 577 (1967).

Buck-Gramcko, D.: Wiederherstellung durchtrennter peripherer Nerven. Chir. Praxis 15, 66 (1971).

Carroll, R. E., Bassett, A. L.: Formation of tendon sheath by silicone-rod implants. J. Bone Joint Surg. A 45, 884 (1963).

Christ, W.: Erfahrungen mit handgelenksnahen Schnittverletzungen. Zentralbl. Chir. 86, 2090 (1961).

Cowan, R. J., Courtemanche, A. D.: An experimental study of tendon suturing techniques. Can. J. Surg. 2, 373 (1959).

Edshage, S.: Peripheral nerve suture. Acta Chir. Scand. [Suppl.] 331, 1 (1964).

Flückiger, R.: De la réparation des tendons fléchisseurs sectionnés au niveau des doigts ("no man's land"). Bern: Dissertation 1964.

Geldmacher, J.: Technik der zweizeitigen freien Beugesehnentransplantation. Handchirurgie 2, 109 (1969).

Hunter, J. M., Salisbury, R. E.: Flexor-tendon reconstruction in severely damaged hand. J. Bone Joint Surg. A 53, 829 (1971).

Kaplan, E. E.: Device for measuring length of tendon graft in flexor tendon surgery of the hand. Bull. Hosp. Joint Dis. 3, 97 (1942).

Koschitz-Kosic, H.: Zum Problem der Narbe bei der Verheilung durchtrennter peripherer Nerven. Langenbecks Arch. Chir. 301, 864 (1962).

Kurtze, T.: Microtechniques in neural surgery. Neurosurgery 11, 128 (1964).

Loew, F.: Die Nervennaht und die Deckung von Nervendefekten bei dem Verschluß akzidenteller und operativ gesetzer Wunden. Chir. Plast. Reconstr. 6, 136 (1969).

Mason, M. C., Allen, H. S.: Rate of healing of tendons, experimental study of tensile strength. Ann. Surg. 113, 424 (1914).

Millesi, H.: Zur Technik der freien Sehnentransplantation. Langenbecks Arch. Chir. 309, 40 (1965).

Mittelmeier, H.: Umscheidungen von Sehnen. Langenbecks Arch. Chir. 304, 938 (1963).

Moberg, E.: Aspects of sensation in reconstructive surgery of the upper extremity. J. Bone Joint Surg. A 46, 817 (1964).

Paneva-Holevich, E.: Two-stage tenoplasty in injuries of the flexor tendons of the hand. J. Bone Joint Surg. A 51, 21 (1969).

Pannike, A., List, M.: Erfahrungen und Wiederherstellungsresultate bei einzeitigem und zweizeitigem Beugesehnenersatz. Monatsschr. Unfallheilkd. 74, 211 (1971).

Pieper, W.: Neuere Operationstechniken in der Beugesehnenchirurgie. Chir. Plast. Reconstr. 6, 13 (1969).

Pulvertaft, R. G.: Tendon grafts for flexor tendon injuries in the fingers and thumb. J. Bone Joint Surg. B 38, 175 (1956).

Pulvertaft, R. G.: Problems of flexor-tendon surgery of the hand. J. Bone Joint Surg. A 47, 123 (1965).

Recht, P.: Frische Nervenverletzungen an der Hand. Langenbecks Arch. Chir. 287, 538 (1957).

Schink, W.: Die Behandlung frischer Sehnenverletzungen. Zentralbl. Chir. 93, 62 (1968).

Seddon, H. J.: The use of autogenous grafts for the repair of large gaps in peripheral nerves. Br. J. Surg. 35, 151 (1966).

Stenström, St. J.: A contribution to the technique of the distal anastomosis in secondary flexor tendon grafting. Plast. Reconstr. Surg. 33, 172 (1964).

Struppler, A.: Myographie in der Facialis- und Handchirurgie. Chir. Plast. Reconstr. 8, 3 (1970).

Tönnis, D.: Der Wert der Elektromyographie für die Beurteilung peripherer Nervenverletzungen. Hefte Unfallheilkd. 81, 312 (1965).

Zrubecky, G.: Plastischer Beugesehnenersatz im Rahmen der chirurgischen Erstversorgung. Monatsschr. Unfallheilkd. 67, 115 (1964).

Zrubecky, G.: Primäre Sehnenplastiken mit der oberflächlichen Beugesehne. Hefte Unfallheilkd. 78, 86 (1964).

Zrubecky, G.: Mitteilung über eine technische Modifikation des primärplastischen Sehnenersatzes an den Langfingern. Monatsschr. Unfallheilkd. 68, 34 (1965).

Capsular Ligament Injuries of the Finger Joints

I. Anatomy

All the interphalangeal joints are of the ginglymoid type. From the center of rotation of the phalangeal heads, the collateral ligaments extend distally to the base of the next bone on each side. Palmarward they become the accessory collateral ligaments, which are not inserted into the bone but radiate to the volar fibrocartilage plate. This plate is broadly fixed at the base of the distal bone, separating the flexor tendon sheath from the articular space, and centralward becomes the thin flaccid pars. The latter is taut during maximum extension and folded in moderate flexion. During maximum flexion it is stretched in a central direction by the rigid fibrocartilage plate. Below the flaccid pars is the volar capsule sac.

The basal, or metacarpophalangeal, joints are of the condyloid type. Their range of motion is limited by a strong ligament system. The lateral ligaments are eccentrically arranged such that they are taut during flexion and somewhat lax during extension (Figure 10a–c). This accounts for the tendency of these joints to stiffen in extension when immobilized in this position.

II. Pathology

Sprains and dislocations as clinical diagnoses find their anatomical substrate in more or less extensive lesions of the capsular ligament apparatus, regardless of the severity of the trauma. Dislocation is always accompanied by a rupture of the capsular ligament, whereas a sprain involves various capsular ligament injuries ranging from strain to laceration. This is sometimes forgotten and can therefore lead to severe functional impairment.

III. Diagnosis

A. Dislocation

The elastic fixation and deformation of the dislocated joint (usually toward the extensor side) are the obvious signs of this condition. An x-ray examination is necessary for documentation purposes and to exclude or confirm accompanying bone injuries. After the dislocation is reduced, the extent of the ligament rupture can be clinically determined by pain and instability and documented by x-rays made under block anesthesia.

"Finger dislocations" in children are often the cause of errors. Epiphysiolysis, rather than joint dislocation, is generally present in such cases.

Dislocations of the distal interphalangeal joints may escape diagnosis due to the "swelling" to which the motor loss is attributed.

X-rays must be made if joint injury is suspected.

B. Sprain (Capsular Ligament Injury Ranging from Strain to Laceration)

The fresh injury is characterized by a painful limitation of motion in the affected joint, combined with a more or less severe fusiform swelling. The pain elicited by pressure and stretching makes it possible to localize the lesion of the capsular ligament. X-ray examination is mandatory. The possible presence of a fine bony avulsion in the joint region makes the "sprained finger joint" a nontrivial injury.

C. Old Capsular Ligament Injuries

The untreated capsular ligament lesion leaves behind a painfully swollen joint with a limited range of motion for some weeks. In the extreme case, the joint become permanently unstable. In ruptures of the ulnar lateral ligament at the basal joint of the thumb or capsular ligament injuries of the saddle joint of the thumb, this can lead to a severe impairment of all natural forms of grasp. Even in long-standing cases, x-ray examination is a useful aid to diagnosis.

Stiffening of the basal joint of the long fingers in extension due to shrinking of the lateral ligaments (resulting from faulty immobilization) must be differentiated from the "intrinsic minus position" due to paralysis.

IV. Treatment

A. Fresh Dorsal Dislocation

Reduction is accomplished under block anesthesia by traction and volar compression against the centrally located phalangeal head. In some cases it will be possible to acheive reduction without anesthesia during the examination, but the patient will be grateful if the physician refrains from reduction without benefit of anesthesia.

After reduction, the part is immobilized in the position of function by means of a plaster cast for 4 weeks. The capsular ligament apparatus must be given the opportunity for undisturbed cicatricial healing.

There are dislocations, of course, that defy closed reduction. They usually involve the basal joints of the thumb and long fingers, and in rare cases the middle joints. In these irreducible dislocations the head of the proximal phalanx protrudes through a rupture of the volar capsular apparatus, and parts of the volar capsular ligament intrude into the joint to hinder its reduction. In the thumb, the tendon of the long flexor muscle may create an absolute obstacle to bloodless reduction. In these cases operative reduction is required. An operation is indicated after the first futile attempt at closed reduction has been made. One is tempted to choose exposure by volar approach, but this raises the danger of iatrogenic injuries. The following procedure is therefore recommended:

1. Long Fingers

The midlateral approach dorsal to the neurovascular bundle is used for the middle joints, and the dorsal approach between the metacarpal heads for the basal joints. The collateral ligaments must be spared. After reduction, suture of the volar capsular ligament apparatus is unnecessary, although the lateral extensor apparatus or interosseous hoods must be reunited by suture if necessary. Immobilization for 4 weeks in the position of function is mandatory.

2. Thumb

The midlateral radial approach to the basal joint is used. Reduction is followed by immobilization in plaster for 5 weeks.

B. Volar Dislocation of the Middle Joint

This type of dislocation is rare and, whether old or recent, requires operative treatment since it is generally accompanied by rupture of a middle slip of the extensor apparatus, and a lateral ligament may act as an absolute obstacle to reduction. Approach is from the dorsal side, and the procedures of extensor tendon surgery are followed (Figure 99).

> **Closed reduction is possible, but function cannot be restored by healing in plaster due to the accompanying rupture of the middle slip of the extensor apparatus.**

C. Old Dorsal Dislocation

Closed reduction may still be possible 8–10 days after the injury; otherwise open reduction is called for. The approach can be made at all three finger joints, as in fresh dislocations. Reduction is followed by immobilization in the position of function for 4 weeks (Figure 96).

D. Fresh Sprain of the Long Finger Joints

The treatment is basically conservative, even if clinical evidence suggests ligament rupture.

> **Operative treatment by ligament suture neither speeds healing nor improves the results.**

The necessary duration of immobilization varies with the extent of the capsular ligament damage: 2–3 weeks are generally sufficient for strains, while at least 4 weeks are required for lacerations. Persistent pain and swelling require a longer period of immobilization.

E. Fresh Sprain of the Basal Joint of the Thumb

In this joint, the complete division of the capsular ligament apparatus must be distinguished from other ligament injuries. Information on the extent of the injury can be obtained by x-ray as well as clinical examination. Rupture of the *ulnar* lateral ligament requires operative treatment if the stability of all natural forms of grasp is to be safely restored. All other ligamentous lesions of the thumb can be treated conservatively.

The basal joint is exposed by a curved ulnar incision. The lateral ligament is sutured with transosseal pull-out wire (Figure 118a,b). The thumb is immobilized in the position of function for 5 weeks in a circular cast that includes the wrist.

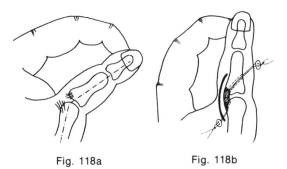

Fig. 118a   Fig. 118b

It is often difficult to convince the patient that this injury must be treated surgically. If the patient categorically rejects surgery, at least an attempt must be made to achieve healing by immobilization in a circular forearm-and-thumb cast for 5 weeks.

F. Inadequately Treated and Old Untreated Capsular Ligament Injuries

Every lesion of the capsular ligament is bridged by scar tissue. This takes time to form. Until this somewhat second-intention healing process is completed, there is a painful limitation of joint motion with swelling. The healing process can be favorably influenced by splinting in the position of function for 4–5 weeks. This generally leads to a complete return to health, even in the case of long-standing injuries.

If the ligament apparatus is ruptured, however, a larger distance must be bridged by scar tissue. This can lead to instability of the joint, and therefore operative measures are required. This applies especially to ruptures of the ulnar lateral ligaments at the basal joint of the thumb. A secondary suture offers little prospect of success in such cases. If no secondary arthrosis is present, an attempt may be made to operatively replace the tendon with the palmar tendon (Figure 119a,b). Even better is a recently publicized reconstructive technique that uses the tendon of the short extensor muscle of the thumb. Otherwise arthrodesis in 160° flexion is preferred. This stabilizes the thumb with no significant loss of function.

The only other joints prone to instability are the middle joints of the long fingers, which may become unstable due to rupture of the collateral ligaments or the capsular ligament connection on the volar side (fibro-cartilage plate, flaccid pars). In this case reattachment or advancement of the ligament apparatus with pull-out wire is advised. After operative treatment, immobilization in a plaster cast for 4 weeks is required.

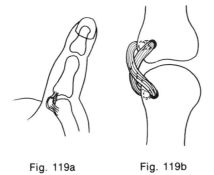

Fig. 119a   Fig. 119b

G. Stiffness of the Basal Joint of the Long Fingers

Excision of the shortened lateral ligaments (capsulectomy) is suitable for improving the mobility of the basal joint. The results of the operation are usually good initially but are not always satisfactory on a long-term basis, even with proper aftercare.

> **Thus, the prophylaxis of stiffness of the basal long finger joints is more important and more successful than its operative treatment.**

The technique of Howard is used: Exposure is by approach from the dorsal side longitudinally through the extensor apparatus or, preferably, between the metacarpal bones. The collateral ligaments are not just severed but also resected, permitting an unobstructed view into the joint (Figure 120a–c).

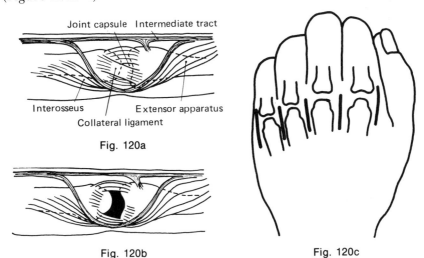

Joint capsule Intermediate tract

Interosseus   Extensor apparatus
Collateral ligament

Fig. 120a

Fig. 120b   Fig. 120c

H. Postoperative Care

The conservative or operative treatment of capsular ligament injuries must be followed by a sufficiently long program of therapeutic exercise under the supervision of the physician and the direction of a physical therapist. The early resumption of ordinary activities will assist in this program. The patient must be advised that, even after proper treatment, complaints may persist for many weeks. The use of an adhesive plaster bandage that prevents extreme articular movements yet allows a sufficient range of motion has proved helpful during the rehabilitative phase at the workplace. It is especially useful for protecting the sensitive middle joints and can easily be applied daily by the patient himself. The joint is fixed in the position of function by 1.25-cm–wide adhesive strips applied longitudinally to the dorsal, volar, radials and ulnar sides of the finger. They are supported by additional diagonal strips. This arrangement is also a good therapeutic measure for mild capsular ligament lesions that have led only to a stretching of the ligament apparatus (Figure 121).

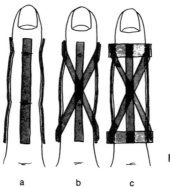

Fig. 121

a   b   c

I. Summary

The conservative treatment of fresh and old capsular ligament injuries of the finger joints is generally preferable to operative treatment, with the following exceptions:

Irreducible dislocations.
Volar dislocations of the middle joints of the long fingers.
Rupture of the ulnar lateral ligament at the basal joint of the thumb.
Old injuries that have led to joint instability.

Stiffening of the basal joint in extension due to shortening of the lateral ligaments.

Bibliography

Curtis, R. M.: Capsulectomy of the interphalangeal joints of the fingers. J. Bone Joint Surg. A 36, 1219 (1254).

Moberg, E.: Fractures and ligamentous injuries of the thumb and fingers. Surg. Clin. North Am. 40, 297 (1960).

Moberg, E., Steuer, B.: Injuries of the ligaments of the thumb and fingers. Diagnosis, treatment and prognosis. Acta Chir. Scand. 106, 166 (1953).

Sakellarides, H. T., DeWeese, J. W.: Instability of the metacarpophalangeal joint of the thumb. Reconstruction of the collateral ligaments using the extensor pollicis brevis tendon. J. Bone Joint Surg. A 58, 106 (1976).

Scharizer, E.: Spätergebnisse von über 300 geschlossenen Bandverletzungen des Daumens. Hefte Unfallheilkd. 78, 88 (1964).

Solonen, K. A.: Rupture of the ulnar collateral ligament of the metacarpophalangeal joint of the thumb. Int. Surg. 45, 669 (1966).

Spinner, M., Choi, B. Y.: Anterior dislocation of the proximal interphalangeal joint. J. Bone Joint Surg. A 52, 1329 (1970).

Witt, A. N.: Funktionsverbessernde Eingriffe an den Fingergelenken. Langenbecks Arch. Chir. 287, 541 (1957).

Fractures of the Phalanges and Metacarpus

The procedure for fractures of the hand follows the same principles that apply generally in the treatment of fractures:

1) Correct diagnosis.
2) Accurate reduction.
3) Sufficiently long immobilization in the position of function.
4) Attention to skin and circulatory conditions.
5) Freedom of movement in all joints except those that *must* be immobilized.

I. Diagnosis

For surgical and forensic reasons, an x-ray examination is an essential part of the diagnostic procedure. It is also indicated if the slightest possibility of bone injury exists. To rely solely on clinical evidence is to place important functions needlessly in jeopardy. Moreover, the squeezing, pulling, and bending of an injured member causes the patient unnecessary pain and should be dispensed with in favor of tests for active joint mobility (functio laesa). Testing for crepitation is obsolete.

In addition to the standard planes, dental films are very useful in the diagnosis of finger joint injuries.

II. Reduction

The kinetic chain from the muscle to the tendon to the tendon insertion is relatively short in the hand region, and even a slight malunion can adversely affect the function of the injured ray by upsetting the muscle balance and, due to the close anatomical and functional relations, may impede the function of the entire hand. The shortening, angulation, and rotational malunion of bones must be avoided. Slight lateral displacements are acceptable. Prolonged traction is an unsuitable technique and promotes distraction and thus pseudoarthrosis. If closed alignment cannot be satisfactorily achieved, open reduction is required. Stable osteosynthesis is also necessary in such cases.

The incision to expose the bone should follow the general principles that apply to incisions, even if it is dictated by wounds.

The result of the reduction is documented by x-ray. Additional films are made 8–10 days later to detect possible secondary redislocations after the initial swelling has subsided and to draw corresponding therapeutic conclusions.

III. Immobilization

As a rule, phalangeal fractures are immobilized in a plaster cast that includes the forearm. Wire or aluminum splints padded with felt or foam rubber are applied to the finger, preferably on the dorsal side. The finger is fixed with adhesive plaster, with the distal phalanx left free. The metacarpal fracture is immobilized in a forearm–fist cast. All immobilized members should be in the position of function.

The duration of immobilization is determined by the clinical and x-ray evidence. In most cases consolidation has progressed so far in 5–6 weeks that the cast can be removed by that time. An exception is the fracture of the shaft of the middle phalanx, which often requires 8 weeks or more. One need not wait for complete bony union as evidenced by the x-rays, since the fracture lines from phalangeal fractures often remain visible for several months.

IV. Surveillance

The extent of a fracture hematoma or post-traumatic edema cannot be calculated in advance. The bandage must therefore be carefully watched for the first few days so that impairments of blood flow can be promptly detected. A constricting bandage must be loosened at once or even replaced. Immediately after primary care is completed, the patient should be told the symptoms of circulatory impairment, especially with

regard to swelling, pain, and discoloration. He must be instructed to notify the physician or nurse at the first sign of such symptoms. The patient
should be alert for "tight spots" and be advised of their possible occurrence. They must be corrected immediately, even if a new bandage
must be applied to do so.

**For forensic reasons, the patient should be requested to acknowledge
these instructions in writing.**

All patients who are treated with a cast at our clinic are asked to sign
the following statement:

CAST STATEMENT

This is to certify that I have been instructed to notify my doctor
or return to the hospital *immediately* at the first sign of pain,
tightness or other discomfort.

Pirmasens,_____(date)

_____
(Signature of patient or guardian)

V. Exercise

The immediate, regular therapeutic exercise of all unimmobilized
joints and members promotes the rapid reduction of swelling and is the
best prophylaxis for dystrophy. The physician must instruct the patient
in the technique of the exercises during primary care and explain the
importance of their regular performance.

In addition to the prompt, supervised exercise of all unimmobilized
joints, it is important that the distal phalanx of the injured digit be left
mobile. This will enable the tendons to glide in the fracture region,
thereby preventing adhesion of the tendon to its sheath or the fracture
and avoiding extensive reconstructive measures or even loss of function.

VI. Care of the Fresh Fracture

A. Fractures of the Distal Phalanx

See the chapter on Fingertip Injuries.

B. Fractures of the Middle and Proximal Phalanges of the Long Fingers

1. Shaft Fractures

As a rule, these fractures are treated conservatively. The typical dislocation is to be noted during reduction: fractures of the proximal phalanx and the proximal two-thirds of the middle phalanx open dorsally due to muscular tension, while fractures of the distal third of the middle phalanx open volarward. After the fracture is reduced under block anesthesia, a plaster cast is applied that includes the forearm and extends to the metacarpophalangeal joints. The finger is fixed in flexion on a well-padded finger splint by means of wide adhesive plaster strips without strangling it. The splint is plastered into the case on the dorsal side (Figure 122).

> The "tongue blade" splint has no place here or anywhere else in hand surgery (Figure 123).

The following are indications for operative treatment:

1) Immediate or secondary redislocation.
2) Compound fractures, especially with concomitant injuries to other important anatomical substrates.
3) Multiple fractures of the phalanges.

Osteosynthesis should be performed during open reduction in order to justify the risk of the operation. Therefore, strict limits should be placed on its indication.

The following are suitable materials for osteosynthesis:

1) Kirschner wires up to 1.4 mm in diameter for transverse and short oblique fractures as well as for comminuted fractures (minimal osteosynthesis).

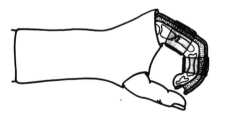
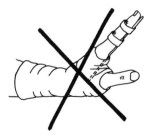

Fig. 122   Fig. 123

2) Wire loops for long oblique and longitudinal fractures.
3) Rush pins for metacarpal fractures.
4) The small-fragment materials of the Association for the Study of Internal Fixation (ASIF).

An oblique incision is made over the dorsal side of the member, turned longitudinally at its distal and proximal ends. The extensor apparatus is slit longitudinally and the fracture is subperiostally exposed (Pratt; Figure 124).

a. Osteosynthesis with Kirschner Wire

The wire is drilled into the distal fragment from the fracture zone such that it emerges at the edge of the finger and its central end disappears in the distal medullary canal. The fracture is then reduced. Fixation is accomplished by retrograde drilling of the wire back into the contralateral cortical substance of the central fragment. The wire is clipped so that its ends disappear beneath the skin (Figure 125). In order to ensure a stable fixation, the angle between the bone and wire axis must be as small as possible without interfering with the adjacent joints. In the short oblique fracture, undesired shortening must be prevented by placing the wire almost vertical to the fracture plane. After the wire is in place, the fragment ends are pressed snugly together.

In comminuted fractures, a Kirschner wire drilled in longitudinally temporarily forms an arthrodesis of the adjacent joints in the position of

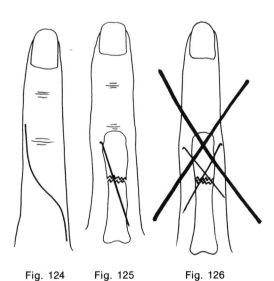

Fig. 124   Fig. 125   Fig. 126

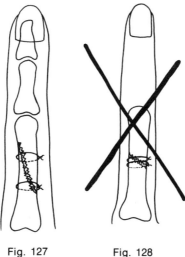

Fig. 127   Fig. 128

function and serves to hold the position of the fracture fragments. It
must be realized that this type of fracture generally leads to partial stiffening. Crossed wires are not recommended in the shaft region, as they
may lead to pseudarthrosis (Figure 126). The wire is removed in 6–8
weeks.

b. Osteosynthesis with Wire Loops

In general, two loops must be applied subperiostally at a sufficient distance from each other to achieve adequate strength (Figure 127). If this
is not possible, the fracture is unsuited for this form of osteosynthesis
(Figure 128). The wires are removed after 6 weeks.

c. Osteosynthesis with ASIF Small-Fragment Screws

This technique can produce excellent results on the proximal phalanx
if employed by an experienced surgeon. Anyone not familiar with the
principles and special technique of the ASIF should resort to one of the
other techniques described above. After osteosynthesis is completed, the
extensor apparatus is united by removable wire suture (Figure 129). The
part is immobilized as in conservative therapy.

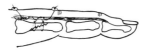

Fig. 129

2. Metaphyseal Fractures with Articular Involvement

A freely mobile, stable, and pain-free joint can be restored only if complete congruence of the articular surfaces can be achieved. As a rule, therefore, it is better to treat joint fractures operatively than conservatively. Even with accurate closed reduction, malunions usually develop later on. The variety of fracture forms that occur (T and Y fractures, shear fractures, and intra-articular condylar fractures) makes it necessary to adapt the exposure and osteosynthetic technique to the conditions at hand (Figures 130–132). Operations of this type are not for the beginner.

Shear fractures can be accurately reduced by exposure through a mid-lateral longitudinal incision, with care being taken to preserve the lateral ligaments. Alternatively, dorsal exposure of the joint by an incision analogous to Pratt's exposure for shaft fractures provides good visibility. Devitalization of the fragments must be avoided if possible, but their complete separation from all soft tissues is no indication for removal. Even in intra-articular condylar fractures the condyles can generally be reunited with the bone.

Osteosynthesis is accomplished with one or more thin (up to 1.0 mm) Kirschner wires, whose placement must be adapted to the situation. Immobilization is as in conservative treatment, and the wires are removed after 6 weeks.

Irreparable interphalangeal joints require primary arthrodesis (Figure 142) to ensure a subsequent painless grasp.

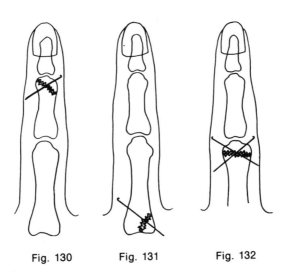

Fig. 130   Fig. 131   Fig. 132

3. Epiphyseal Separation

This separation requires accurate reduction to prevent disturbances of growth and is generally amenable to conservative treatment. If an epiphysiolysis cannot be held in plaster, drill-wire osteosynthesis is permitted. In this case the wire should cross the epiphyseal plate at a right angle if possible, simultaneously creating a temporary arthrodesis.

C. Fractures of the Thumb

1. Fractures of the Distal Phalanx

See the chapter on Fingertip Injuries.

2. Shaft Fractures of the Proximal Phalanx

Conservative treatment in a circular plaster case is indicated. It holds the thumb in the position of function, includes the metacarpus and forearm, and allows free mobility of the long fingers. The thumb tip must remain visible (Figure 20).

An indication for operative treatment is seldom present, at least in closed fractures, because mild dislocations usually pose no threat to function.

3. Sesamoid Fractures

These fractures temporarily cause a painful limitation of motion and are therefore immobilized for 1 week in a dorsal forearm–thumb cast before mobility is restored by exercise.

4. Articular Fractures

Articular fractures of the long fingers are treated operatively. They are an indication for primary arthrodesis. Arthrodesis can be applied more liberally, because the basal joint in particular requires stability more than mobility in order to ensure thumb function (Figures 91b, 142).

D. Fractures of the Second through Fifth Metacarpals

Metacarpal fractures can impede the grasping function of the entire hand as the result of shortening, angulation, or rotational malunion. It is difficult to standardize the treatment of such fractures, however, due to

their great morphological variety. Closed reduction is of limited value
due to the close spacial and functional relations among adjacent bones.
Even a successful reduction may be ruined by the often large fracture
hematoma which develops on the dorsum of the hand and prevents adequate fixation of the bone in the case. It is little wonder that percutaneous and other forms of osteosynthesis have been employed in this area
for some time. Two disadvantages of this technique must not be overlooked, however: (1) an accurate reduction and functionally stable osteosynthesis are seldom achieved by this method and (2) the iatrogenic injury of functionally important anatomical structures in the basal joint
region is often unavoidable, quite apart from a blockage of the joint,
which requires lengthy postoperative treatment after the bone has
healed. Osteosynthesis is useless if it increases the risks of treatment
without yielding functional benefits.   Osteosynthesis with the plate and
screw implants of the ASIF offers a way out of these difficulties (Figure
133). However, this technique requires an experienced surgeon as well
as the special instruments of the ASIF.

Despite the difficulties indicated, we shall attempt to lay down some
generally valid guidelines for routine practice:

1) Stable metacarpal fractures are treated conservatively for 4–6
weeks in a forearm–fist cast (analogous to Figure 159). These include
most basal fractures as well as transverse fractures with only a slight lateral displacement. After the cast is applied, x-ray films must be made to
document the results of the reduction and to determine whether the
basal joints of the long fingers are adequate flexed.

2) Even closed, unstable metacarpal fractures may be treated conservatively after closed reduction. The alignment is made as accurately as
possible under block anesthesia, followed by fixation for 5–8 weeks in a

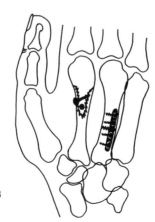

Fig. 133

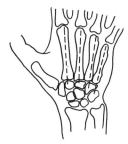

Fig. 134

forearm–fist cast. Rotational malunions and the consequent overlapping of fingers when the fist is closed can be safely prevented by this method. The slight decrease in bone length that may occur in oblique fractures generally impairs only the appearance of the hand, but not its function. If angulations and significant shortenings go uncorrected, they lead to functional disability by destroying the muscle balance. They therefore require at least an approximate anatomical reduction combined with osteosynthesis. This can be done with certainty only in the open wound. The fractured metacarpal is exposed by an incision parallel to the metacarpal axis, with care being taken to handle the tendons atraumatically (Figure 134). Open fractures are not a contraindication to operative treatment.

3)   Open reduction without osteosynthesis does not ensure retention of the fracture fragments. It only increases the risks of treatment without increasing the functional gain. This procedure therefore is not recommended.

4)   The osteosynthesis must be sufficiently stable to maintain alignment, at least with the aid of the fist cast, which is indicated in most forms of wire osteosynthesis. A stability sufficient for exercise can be achieved only by fixation with plates and screws.

5)   When the osteosynthesis material is implanted, care must be taken that the function of the metacarpophalangeal joints is not impaired and no secondary injuries are incurred.

6)   Crossed Kirschner wires are appropriate only in the case of metaphyseal fractures. In shaft fractures, they could lead to pseudarthrosis (Figure 135). The latter type of fracture requires fixation with an oblique drill wire by the method of Pratt (Figure 125), retrograde intermedullary splinting by the method of Iselin (Figure 136a,b), or lashing with wire loops (Figure 127).

7)   The often extensive fracture hematoma on the dorsum in the subaponeurotic space must be drawn off by suction drainage in a sterile closed system (Redon). This is true not only for operative treatment; conservative treatment may also require removal of the hematoma by a

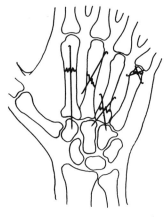

Fig. 135

suction drain introduced through a puncture incision under highly
aseptic conditions in order to maintain the alignment by accurate immobilization.

E. Fractures of the First Metacarpal

The same principles apply as for the other metacarpal bones. The
hand is immobilized in the position of function by means of a circular
forearm–thumb cast that includes the metacarpus but allows the metacarpophalangeal joints of the long fingers full freedom of motion.

Of the fractures near the base of the bone, Bennet's fracture–dislocation (Figure 137) merits special attention. A persistent dislocation or subluxation as well as the inadequate repair of the articular surface at the
base of the first metacarpal can lead to a severe, highly painful functional impairment of the saddle joint and thus of grasping in general.

Alignment is easily accomplished: By pulling on the abducted and
semiopposed thumb and applying external pressure on the base of the
first metacarpal, the physician can almost always achieve a satisfactory

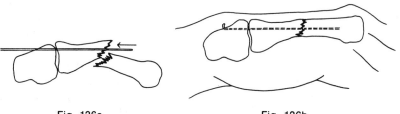

Fig. 136a   Fig. 136b

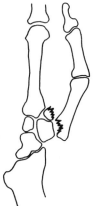
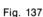

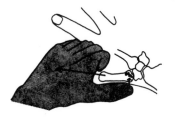

Fig. 137   Fig. 138

alignment (Figure 138). Prolonged plaster fixation is seldom successful, however, because the circular forearm–thumb cast applied under the conditions of the reduction maneuver cannot prevent redislocation due to the thick mantle of soft tissue. We therefore remain conservative only in exceptional cases, consider percutaneous drill-wire osteosynthesis problematic, and prefer open reduction combined with drill-wire osteosynthesis. Exposure is achieved by the method of Wagner (Figure 139) or of Moberg and Gedda (Figure 140). After anatomical reduction, the small basal fragment is engaged with a 1-mm Kirschner wire introduced through the first metacarpal. If the fragment is very small, the wire can be drilled into the multangulum majus. To improve the stability of the osteosynthesis, the first metacarpal is fixed in opposition to the second

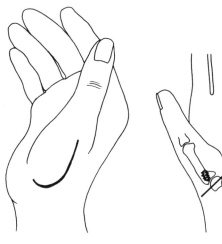

Fig. 139   Fig. 140

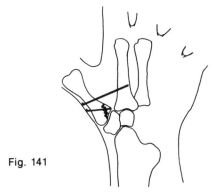

Fig. 141

metacarpal with the second wire (Figure 141). Immobilization in plaster is recommended as an adjunctive measure. The possibility of a functionally stable osteosynthesis using small-fragment screws (Burri, Willebrand) is mentioned in passing.

VII. Repair of Malunited Finger and Metacarpal Fractures, Pseudarthrosis, and Tendon Blocks after Fractures

These operations require considerable technical skill. It must be determined beforehand whether the potential gain outweighs the risk and whether one's own surgical skills are sufficient to cope with atypical situations. The special case of the first ray is discussed in the chapter on Thumb Injuries.

A. Fractures with Articular Involvement

1. Indications

Stiffening in an unfavorable position and a joint that gives pain on motion are indications for operation.

2. Technique

a. Interphalangeal Joints

An arthrodesis is created in a favorable position of flexion, generally about 135° (Figure 142a–c).

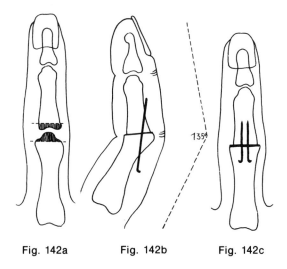

Fig. 142a   Fig. 142b   Fig. 142c

b. Metacarpophalangeal Joints

Resection of the metacarpal head (Figure 143a,b) or arthroplasty (Figure 144a,b) is performed. We prefer simple resection.

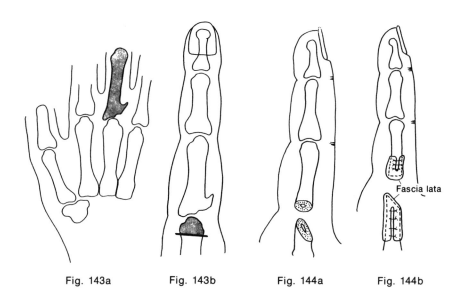

Fig. 143a   Fig. 143b   Fig. 144a   Fig. 144b

B. Shaft Fractures of the Middle and Proximal Phalanges

1. Indications

Gross incapacitating malunions, especially angulations, that impair the muscle balance are indications for operation. Restraint is advised for purely cosmetic indications.

2. Technique

a. *Angulation*

Cuneiform osteotomy (Figure 145a,b), alignment by insertion of an autologous bone graft from the iliac crest (Figure 146a,b), or drill-wire osteosynthesis is performed.

b. *Rotational Malunion*

For the middle phalanx, derotational osteotomy with drill-wire osteosynthesis is performed (only rarely indicated as functional gain is problematic). For the proximal phalanx, derotational osteotomy near the base of the associated metacarpal or drill-wire osteosynthesis is performed.

c. *Shortening*

Lengthening osteotomy with insertion of an autologous bone graft is performed (very rarely indicated as functional gain is problematic and there is danger of ischemia).

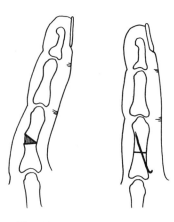

Fig. 145a   Fig. 145b

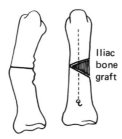

Fig. 146a   Fig. 146b

C. Metacarpal Fractures

The indications and reconstructive measures follow the same principles that apply in fractures of the phalanges. The indications for a lengthening osteotomy are somewhat broader.

D. Pseudarthrosis

1. Indications

A flaccid false joint, a rigid false joint only if it causes pain or impairs function, and defect pseudarthrosis are indications for operation. It should be noted that after severe injuries with partial stiffening of the fingers, a pseudarthrosis may painlessly assume the lost functions.

2. Technique

Union by autologous bone graft is performed (Figure 147a–c).

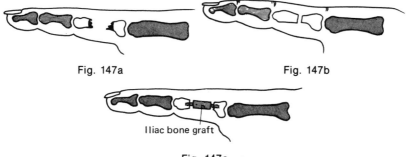

Fig. 147a   Fig. 147b

Iliac bone graft

Fig. 147c

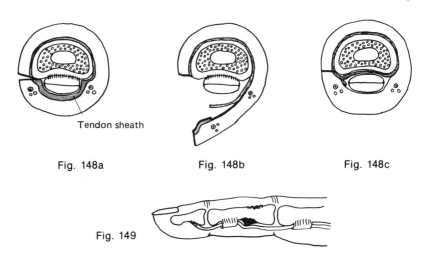

Fig. 148a   Fig. 148b   Fig. 148c

Fig. 149

E. Tendon Block

1. Indications

Destruction of the sheath and adherence to the fracture callus, excessive callus formation and avulsed fragments which lead to impaired muscle balance.

2. Technique

a. Tendon Adhesions

Tendolysis is performed; a pedicled fat graft can be used to block the tendon on the dorsal side, while the tendon sheath can be used on the volar side (Figure 148a–c). The success of these measures can be judged only after intensive therapeutic exercise but they often remain problematic.

b. Bony Protuberances with Impairment of Muscle Balance

Restoration of natural bone contours is accomplished by ablation of protuberances, combined with tendolysis if necessary. The prognosis is better than in the case of tendon adhesions (Figure 149).

Bibliography

Beckenbough, R. D., Dobyns, J. H., Linscheid, R. L., Bryan, R. S.: Review and analysis of silicone rubber metacarpophalangeal implants. J. Bone Joint Surg. A 58, 483 (1976).

Berkman, E. F., Miles, G. H.: Internal fixation of metacarpal fracture exclusive of the thumb. J. Bone Joint Surg. 24, 816 (1943).

Brandt, G.: Die wesentlichen Gesichtspunkte für die Behandlung der geschlossenen Frakturen im Bereich von Finger und Hand. Langenbecks Arch. Chir. 287, 498 (1957).

Brody, G. S., White, W. L.: New concepts in prosthetic joints for use in the hand. Plast. reconstr. Surg. 32, 45 (1963).

Buck-Gramcko, D.: Funktionsverbessernde Eingriffe an den Fingergelenken. Chir. plast. Reconstr. 7, 44 (1970).

Burri, C., et al.: Stabile Osteosynthese. Frakturen im Handbereich. Aktuelle Chir. 4, 305 (1969).

Crawford, G. P.: Screw fixation for certain fractures of the phalanges and metacarpals. J. Bone Joint Surg. A 58, 487 (1976).

Eades, J. W., Peacock, E. E.: Autogenous transplantation of an interphalangeal joint and proximal phalangeal epiphysis. J. Bone Joint Surg. A 48, 775 (1966).

Flatt, A. E.: Fracture–dislocations of an index metacarpophalangeal joint and an ulnar deviating force in the flexor tendons. J. Bone Joint Surg. A 48, 100 (1966).

Fowler, G. B.: Mobilisation of metacarpophalangeal joint. J. Bone Joint Surg. 29, 193 (1947).

Gedda, K. O.: Studies on Bennet's fracture. Anatomy, roentgenology and therapy. Acta Chir. Scand. [Suppl.] 193 (1954).

Janss, S. A.: Fractures of the metacarpal. A new method of reduction and immobilisation. J. Bone Joint Surg. 20, 178 (1938).

Littler, J. W.: Metcarpal reconstruction. J. Bone Joint Surg. 29, 723 (1947).

Lungmus, F.: Die Sesambeinbrüche des Daumens. Monatsschr. Unfallheilkd. 56, 233 (1953).

Mansoor, J. A.: Metacarpal lengthening. A case report. J. Bone Joint Surg. A 51, 1638 (1969).

Nicolai, N.: Die operative Behandlung der Fingerpseudarthrosen. Langenbecks Arch. Chir. 299, 135 (1961).

Pratt, D. R.: Exposing fractures of the proximal phalanx of the finger longitudinally through the dorsal extensor apparatus. In: De Palma, A. F. (ed.): Clinical orthopaedics, Vol. 15. Philadelphia: Lippincott 1959.

Swanson, A. B.: Silicone rubber implants for replacement of arthritic or destroyed joints of the hand. Surg. Clin. North Am. 48, 1113 (1968).

Thevenin, R.: L'appareil standard réduit pour l'immobilisation des fractures des phalanges. Chir. Main (Paris) 12, 40 (1970).

Wagner, C. J.: Method of treatment of Bennett's fracture dislocation. Am. J. Surg. 80, 230 (1950).

Wainwright, D.: Fractures of the metacarpals and phalanges. Proc. R. Soc. Med. 57, 598 (1964).

Waugh, R. L., Ferrozzano, G. P.: Fractures of the metacarpal exclusive of the thumb. A new method of treatment. Am. J. Surg. 59, 186 (1943).

Weckesser, E. G.: Rotational osteotomy of the metacarpal for overlapping fingers. J. Bone Joint Surg. A 47, 751 (1965).

Willebrand, H., Schweikert, Ch.: Läßt sich die Versorgung der Mittelhandfrakturen standardisieren? Chir. Plast. Reconstr. 6, 43 (1969).

Zrubecky, G., Keller, B.: Operative Behandlung und plastischer Ersatz von versteiften Mittelgelenken. Chir. Praxis 4, 69 (1960).

Fractures and Dislocations
of the Carpal Bones

I. General

For anatomical reaons, fractures of the carpal bones are relatively unfavorable in terms of their healing tendency. They are difficult to immobilize with precision, and their healing can be delayed or prevented by
the devitalization of a fragment. This is especially true of scaphoid fractures.

Any carpal bone can be fractured by direct trauma. Indirect traumas
lead mainly to fractures of the scaphoid and lunate, as well as to dislocations and fracture–dislocations, which must be considered in connection
with pure carpal fractures for diagnostic and therapeutic reasons.

Scaphoid fractures are by far the most common of the carpal fractures, while dislocations and fracture–dislocations of this bone are rare.
This is no excuse for overlooking such injuries, however, due to their
marked effects on wrist function.

Pain or morphological changes in the wrist region (Figure 150) following a direct or indirect trauma to the wrist thus require a thorough x-ray
examination in addition to the clinical examination, which must include
tests for neuropathy (lunate dislocation). The proper evaluation of carpal x-rays takes time. A "diagnosis at a glance" is often incorrect.

Films taken in the standard planes are not always sufficient, especially
in fractures of the scaphoid, hamate, and pisiform. If x-ray evidence is
negative while a clinical suspicion is present, preliminary immobilization
of the wrist by means of a dorsal plaster splint that extends from the
metacarpophalangeal joints to the elbow is always correct.

A follow-up x-ray examination after 2 weeks often reveals a fracture
due to the intervening resorptive expansion of the fracture line.

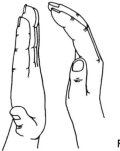

Fig. 150

II. Special X-ray Diagnostics

A. Scaphoid Bone

1. Scaphoid Standard Series

1) The wrist is sagittal with the fist closed, thereby placing the scaphoid parallel to the film plane [a "triangular lunate" is indicative of a lunate dislocation (Figure 151)].
2) The wrist is frontal with fist closed; this view also shows dislocations in the lunate region.
3) The wrist is viewed with the fist closed and the forearm supinated 15°–20° to reveal transverse fractures of the proximal third.

2. Additional X-ray Techniques

1) A rotation series of the wrist is taken with the fist closed in 50°, 60°, 70°, and 80° supination to reveal vertical oblique fractures of the proximal half of the scaphoid.
2) Laminagrams aid not only in difficult diagnoses, but especially in judging the success of treatment.

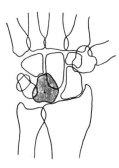

Fig. 151

3) Magnified or fine-focus photographs are an aid in determining the extent of fracture healing, but appear to be dispensible in view of the greater accuracy of laminagraphy.

B. Central Carpal X-rays by the Method of Hart-Gaynor and Barthold to Visualize the Carpal Canal and Canal of Guyon

Tangential films are made of the wrist in extreme dorsiflexion in the intermediate position as well as with the hand rotated 45° ulnarward and radialward (Figure 152). These views reveal changes in the region of the lunate as well as injuries of the hamate and pisiform (Figure 153a–c).

III. Treatment

A. Fresh Scaphoid Fracture, Delayed Scaphoid Union, and Scaphoid Pseudarthrosis

A basic distinction must be made between intra-articular fractures of the body of the scaphoid bone and extra-articular fractures of its tuberosity. The latter are problem free and generally heal completely within 3 months when treated with a dorsal cast that extends from the metacarpophalangeal joints to the elbow.

Several points must be remembered in the treatment of the intra-articular scaphoid fracture:

1) Fractures of the central third of the scaphoid require longer immobilization than more distally located fractures. This has to do with the vascularization of these areas. The 10- to 12-week immobilization recommended by Böhler for central fractures probably represents the lower limit for this category of fractures, as does the 6–8 weeks for fractures of the distal thirds.

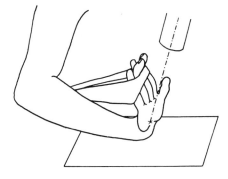

Fig. 152

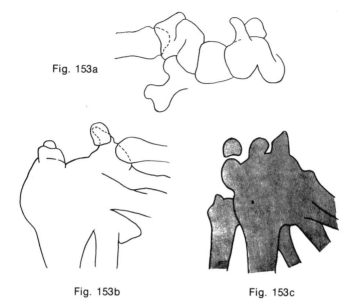

Fig. 153a

Fig. 153b   Fig. 153c

2) Compressive, tangential, and bending forces act on the scaphoid fracture fragments in a manner analogous to the conditions at the neck of the femur. We thus distinguish the following fracture forms:

a) Horizontal oblique fractures (corresponding to Pauwels I; Figure 154a,b).
b) Transverse fractures (corresponding to Pauwels II; Figure 155a,b).
c) Vertical oblique fractures (corresponding to Pauwels III; Figure 156a–c).

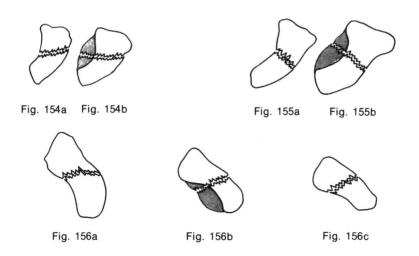

Fig. 154a   Fig. 154b   Fig. 155a   Fig. 155b

Fig. 156a   Fig. 156b   Fig. 156c

The form of the fracture has a marked effect on its consolidation time. Vertical oblique fractures are more likely to produce pseudarthrosis than are horizontal oblique fractures.

1. Should the Fresh Intra-articular Scaphoid Fracture be Treated Operatively or Conservatively?

The polarity of this question can impose directions on the therapy of scaphoid fractures that may work to the patient's disadvantage. There is no question that primary osteosynthesis of the scaphoid can produce excellent functional results without prolonged immobilization if it is truly stable and does not promote the devitalization of a fragment. The ASIF has developed instruments and metal implants for use in osteosynthesis, but this is a technique best left to the experienced surgeon (Figure 157). Minimal osteosynthesis with Kirschner wires is not advised (Figure 158). There is also no doubt that purely conservative treatment with plaster fixation can effect the complete healing of most scaphoid fractures.

We should thus formulate the previous question somewhat differently:

2. How Long Should the Fresh Intra-articular Scaphoid Fracture be Treated Conservatively, and at What Point Should Operative Treatment Begin?

Basically, every scaphoid fracture should be treated conservatively as long as no pseudarthrosis has developed. However, pseudarthrosis may

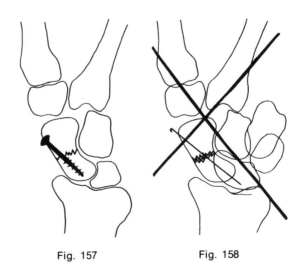

Fig. 157   Fig. 158

appear months or even years after the accident. For psychological and economic reasons, a patient can no longer be expected to tolerate such a lengthy immobilization. Nonetheless, conservative treatment is entirely reasonable up to the 12th week. If the x-ray then shows no healing or at least a healing tendency in the form of a revitalized proximal fragment, the union is "delayed," and the time for operative intervention has arrived.

Whether screw osteosynthesis (ASIF) or a bone graft (Matti, Russe) is employed depends on the local circumstances and the experience of the surgeon. As the biological technique, the bone graft is preferred. We have obtained poor results with screw osteosynthesis when the central fragment was devitalized, even if it was large enough to ensure stable placement of the screw. We have therefore abandoned this technique.

3. Conservative Treatment of the Fresh Scaphoid Fracture

a. *Indications*

All fresh scaphoid fractures without gross dislocation should be treated conservatively.

b. *Technique*

A forearm–fist cast is applied for 12 weeks in the following position: elbow joint in 100° flexion, writing position, and dorsal flexion of the wrist with radial abduction; only the fingertips remain free (Düben and Rehbein, Verdan, Weller; Figure 159). If swelling is severe, it is best to apply only a dorsal plaster splint for the first 10 days instead of splitting the cast.

After the cast is removed, the joints regain their full mobility in a remarkably short time.

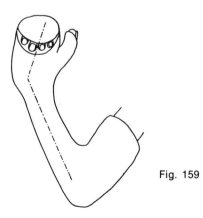

Fig. 159

4. Operative Treatment of the Scaphoid Fracture by
   Bone Grafting and Styloidectomy

a. *Indications*

Scaphoid delayed union after the 12th week, pseudarthrosis, and
fresh scaphoid fractures with gross dislocation are indications for surgery.

b. *Contraindications*

Surgery should not be performed in cases of secondary arthrosis of
the wrist associated with old pseudarthrosis.

c. *Technique*

McLaughlin's approach is recommended for exposure of the scaphoid
and radiocarpal joint (Figure 160). The scaphoid is exposed by a curved
transverse capsular incision near the radius with the wrist in 30° volar
flexion and maximum ulnar abduction. In this way the vascular supply
of the scaphoid is largely preserved. The fracture zone is cleaned with a
small fraise. A socket is made in each fracture fragment for receiving the
bone graft—a chip of cancellous and cortical tissue cut from the styloid
process of the radius (Figure 161). Any remaining gaps can be filled
from the large cancellous reservoir at the lower end of the radius.

Wilhelm's technique of the central scaphoid graft, which requires special instruments, is mentioned in passing.

Whether the occasionally recommended styloidectomy is sufficient in
itself for the treatment of the delayed-union scaphoid fracture remains
an open question. In the final analysis, however, the styloidectomy is a
half-way measure that cannot safely ensure bony union (Verdan).

Postoperative immobilization is required for *at least* 8–10 weeks in a
long arm cast. For manual laborers, a fulled leather sleeve with a steel
splint insert is prescribed for the first year after the resumption of work.

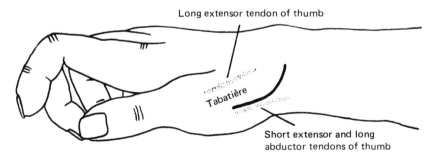

Fig. 160

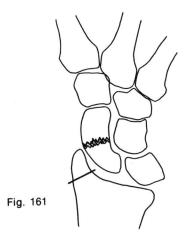

Fig. 161

It extends from the metacarpophalangeal joints to the elbow but leaves the long fingers and thumb entirely free to move. A similar sleeve made of semiflexible plastic is unsuitable because it does not absorb skin moisture during work and thus leads to skin lesions.

The rare cases in which the fresh scaphoid fracture is accompanied by gross dislocation should be treated by open reduction as well as screw osteosynthesis.

A small devitalized central fragment is best removed. This can easily be accomplished from the original incision.

5. Pseudarthrosis of the Scaphoid versus
   Naviculare Bipartitum

A misdiagnosis can have considerable consequences in terms of patient insurance. Recall that true scaphoid pseudarthrosis may produce no symptoms for years, even though it has led to secondary arthrosis of the wrist, and may suddenly become manifest as the result of trauma. On the other hand, the absence of degenerative changes of the wrist does not necessarily indicate naviculare bipartitum. In the final analysis, scaphoid pseudarthrosis can be reliably distinguished from naviculare bipartitum only on the basis of a subtle anamnesis, clinical evidence, and if necessary, observation of the progress of the condition.

B. Fractures of the Other Carpal Bones

The other carpal bones are so firmly seated in the wrist that gross fragment dislocations are uncommon, and these fractures generally heal completely in a forearm–fist cast in 4–8 weeks. Fractures of the lunate bone merit particular attention, as the fracture may become displaced volarward, compressing the carpal canal and producing a median compression syndrome (Figure 162). Also of importance are fractures of the hamulus of the hamate and of the pisiform (Figure 163a,b), which may result in damage to the ulnar nerve in Guyon's canal. These fractures require operative decompression of the nerve by removal of the fracture fragments. Combined injuries involving other carpal bones also occur, such as the concurrent fracture of the scaphoid and capitate.

C. Dislocations and Fracture–Dislocations

These are rare but serious injuries that are caused by indirect trauma and tend to occur as intercarpal dislocations in the region of the lunate. The prognosis of these injuries depends both on the timing of the reduction and on the extent of accompanying capsular ligament damage; by comparison, fractures play a secondary role (Motta). Radiocarpal dislocations are quite rare. A pronounced rarity is the isolated, radialward dislocation of the scaphoid, as well as the "naviculocapitate fracture syn-

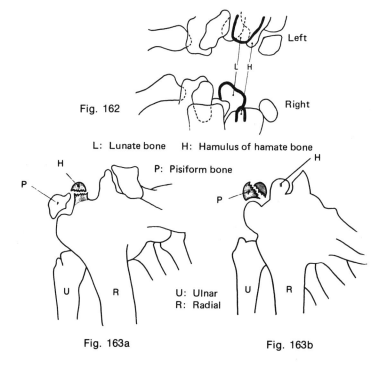

Fig. 162

Left

Right

L: Lunate bone   H: Hamulus of hamate bone

P: Pisiform bone

U: Ulnar
R: Radial

Fig. 163a   Fig. 163b

drome" (Fenton, Marsh and Jones): transverse fracture of the scaphoid (navicular) combined with transverse fracture of the capitate in the proximal third, with the central capitate fragment rotated 180° and displaced palmarward. The clinical picture corresponds to that of a wrist sprain.

The following injuries are most common:

1) Volarward dislocation of the lunate (Figures 151, 164a,b). (Note that the dislocated lunate appears triangular in the anteroposterior film.)
2) Perilunar dislocation, usually dorsalward and rarely palmarward, often combined with styloid fractures (Figure 165).
3) Perinaviculolunar dislocation (Figure 166).
4) Transnaviculolunar dislocation (Figure 167).
5) Transnaviculotranslunar dislocation (Figure 168).
6) Peritriquetrolunar dislocation (Figure 169).

Clinically, the isolated lunate dislocation can sometimes be felt between the thenar and hypothenar. In the other injuries, the diagnosis is

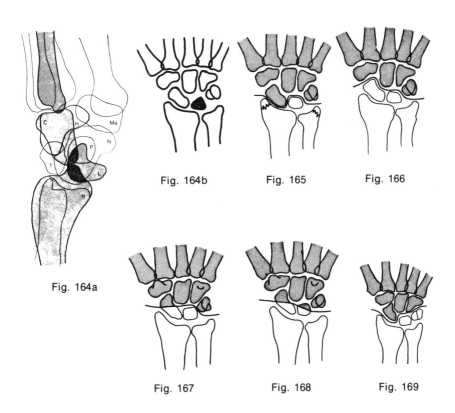

Fig. 164b   Fig. 165   Fig. 166

Fig. 164a

Fig. 167   Fig. 168   Fig. 169

made on the basis of the fork-like position of the hand with a shortened carpus, an obliterated tabatière and the inability to close the fist. This diagnosis must be confirmed by x-ray (Figure 150).

1. Fresh Dislocations and Fracture–Dislocations

Böhler advises 10–15 minutes of steady horizontal or vertical traction under anesthesia. This will free the posterior horn of the lunate from the capitate and allow closed reduction. Gentle manual pressure can assist in the reduction maneuver, although in the isolated lunate dislocation great caution is advised so as not to damage the median nerve, which is drawn tight over the lunate. Dislocations are immobilized in a fist cast for an additional 4 weeks, while fracture–dislocations are treated according to the rules for the treatment of carpal fractures in a long arm cast until consolidation is achieved.

If the reduction is not stable, the carpus is also fixed to the radius with two Kirschner wires.

2. Old Dislocations and Fracture–Dislocations

After the third week, closed reduction is seldom successful. Nevertheless, it should be attempted in view of the risks of open reduction. If an operation proves necessary, the approach is made from the dorsal side (Figure 170a), unless of course a volar approach is warranted by signs of median nerve compression (Figure 170b). The incision must conform to the basic principles of hand surgery.

Perilunar dislocations and fracture–dislocations are always reduced operatively, with varying anatomical results. The lunate dislocation, on the other hand, may defy all reduction maneuvers, even operative ones. The prognosis of the isolated extirpation of the lunate, which is recommended by many authors in such cases, and the concurrent two-thirds resection of the scaphoid bone should be viewed with very cautious optimism with regard to the functional outcome.

D. Carpal Injuries and Arthrodesis of the Wrist

A mobile, pain-free wrist that can be actively stabilized is essential for normal hand function. A painful wrist may lead to considerable disability. However, a wrist that is stiff yet pain free will not deprive the hand of most of its functions owing to the compensatory ability of the shoulder

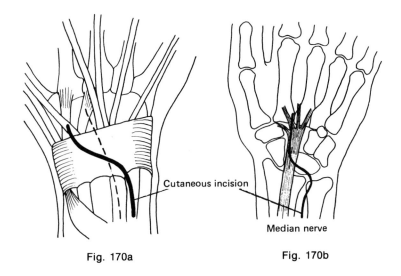

Cutaneous incision

Median nerve

Fig. 170a   Fig. 170b

joint. Hence, the maintenance of wrist mobility is feasible only if a pain-less grasp is ensured. The wrist should thus be considered a "second-order" joint whose operative stiffening may be desirable.

1. Indications for Wrist Arthrodesis

Wrist arthrodesis is indicated in severe arthrosis with a painful limita-tion of wrist motion that impairs the function of the entire hand. This applies especially to pains caused by old scaphoid pseudarthrosis and old lunate dislocations, as well as to pains following wrist infections and intra-articular comminuted fractures of the lower end of the radius. Wil-helm's denervation offers a less radical alternative to this method.

2. Technique for Radiocarpal Arthrodesis

An incision curved toward the ulnar side is made on the dorsum of the wrist (Figure 171a). The extensor tendons are pushed aside ulnarward. The radiocarpal joint is freed of cartilage at a dorsally open angle. The exposed bone surfaces are apposed, and the gap is bridged with a trian-gular bone graft from the dorsal surface of the radius which is inserted into the capitate in a precut groove (Figure 171b). Immobilization in a long arm cast is required until bony union is achieved, which generally takes 12 weeks.

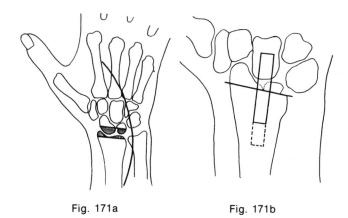

Fig. 171a   Fig. 171b

E. Lunatomalacia (Kienböck's Disease):
   Is It a Sequel to Injury?

   This condition is expressed clinically in pains in the wrist area, and the x-ray shows a densification of the bone as evidence of osteonecrosis. The cause of this condition is still disputed, but it is no longer justified to reject a traumatic causation in every case, especially in view of the fact that lunate fractures may escape x-ray diagnosis in the living subject (Lang, Mordeja). It appears that the development of lunatomalacia requires not a severe trauma, but an *appropriate* one.

   According to Maurer and Lechner, the following are evidence for a traumatic causation:

1) An appropriate traumatic event (a fall on the outstretched hand, severe contusion of the wrist).
2) Clinical manifestations shortly after the accident (pain, swelling, motor impairment).
3) Evidence of a fissure of fracture immediately after the accident or within the first 3–4 weeks.
4) Normal x-ray evidence immediately after the accident and the onset of osteonecrosis no sooner than 4 weeks after the accident; progression of malacic processes.
5) Bridging symptoms between the accident and the evaluation.
6) Absence of a form variant (especially the minus variant of the ulna) and absence of arthrotic changes.

   The following are evidence against a traumatic causation:

1) Changes visible in x-ray that predate the accident, and the appearance of malacia before the fifth week after the accident.

2) Questionable trauma (sprain of the wrist or "strain").
3) Lack of change in x-ray films.
4) Form variants.
5) Bilateral occurrence of the disease.

> **In view of the possible consequences in terms of insurance benefits, the physician is reminded of the importance of x-ray examination even in trivial injuries of the wrist.**

Bibliography

Adler, J. B., Shafton, G. W.: Fractures of the capitate. J. Bone Joint Surg. A 44, 1537 (1962).

Backmann, L., Sassa, W.: Differentialdiagnose der Spaltbildungen des Kahnbeins der Hand, Chir. Praxis 14, 83 (1970).

Bayer, F.: Os naviculare bipartitum. Z. Anat. 103, 634 (1934).

Böhler, L., et al.: Behandlungsergebnisse von 734 frischen einfachen Brüchen des Kahnbeinkörpers der Hand. In: Wiederherstellungschirurgie und Tramatologie, Vol. 2. Basel-New York: Karger 1954.

Brückner, H.: Die Verrenkung des 1. Handstrahles mitsamt dem großen Vieleckbein und Kahnbein. Monatsschr. Unfallheilkd. 65, 398 (1962).

Campbell, R. D., Lange, E. M., Yeah, C. B.: Lunate and perilunar dislocation. J. Bone Joint Surg. B 46, 55 (1964).

Campbell, R. D., et al.: Indications for open reduction of lunate and perilunate dislocation of the carpal joint. J. Bone Joint Surg. A 47, 915 (1965).

Coleman, H. M.: Injuries of the articular disc at the wrist. J. Bone Joint Surg. B 42, 522 (1961).

Düben, W.: Zur Frage der operativen oder konservativen Faustgipsbehandlung des veralteten Kahnbeinbruches und der -pseudarthrosen. Chirurg 25, 63 (1954).

Düben, W., Rehbein, F.: Zur konservativen Behandlung der veralteten Kahnbeinbrüche und der Kahnbeinpseudarthrose. Arch. Orthop. Unfallchir. 45, 67 (1952).

Fenton, R. L.: The naviculo-capitate fracture syndrome. J. Bone Joint Surg. A 37, 681 (1956).

Fleischer, H.: Die autoplastische Spongiosaeinpflanzung bei Kahnbeinpseudarthrosen. Langenbecks Arch. Chir. 309, 68 (1965).

Franke, K.: Über Handgelenksluxationen. Zentralbl. Chir. 89, 1298 (1964).

Gordon, L. H., King, D.: Partial wrist arthrodesis for old ununited fractures of the carpal navicular. Am. J. Surg. 102, 460 (1961).

Grashey, R.: Echte und scheinbare Mondbeinfraktur. Röntgenpraxis 8, 243 (1936).

Immermann, E. W.: Dislocation of the pisiform. J. Bone Joint Surg. A. 30, 489 (1948).

Koch, W., Selentin, W.: Die übersehene perilunäre Luxation. Chirurg 40, 132 (1969).

Malone, L. A.: Post traumatic cystic disease of the carpal bones. Am. J. Roentgenol. 29, 612 (1933).

Matti, H.: Über freie Transplantation von Knochenspongiosa. Arch. Klin. Chir. 168, 236 (1932).

Maurer, G.: Begutachtung der Lunatummalazie. Langenbecks Arch. Chir. 298, 414 (1960).

Mordeja, J.: Eine Abart der intercarpalen Luxationsfraktur:transnaviculotranslunäre dorsale Handluxation. Monatsschr. Unfallheilkd. 65, 200 (1962).

Motta, C.: Spätergebnisse der perilunären Handgelenksverrenkung. Monatsschr. Unfall-heilkd. 65, 377 (1962).

Niederecker, K.: Operative Behandlung schlecht geheilter Knochenbrüche im Bereich des Handgelenkes. Verh. Dtsch. Orthop. Ges., 43, Kongr. 1955, p. 205.

Nusselt, St.: Radiale Kahnbeinverrenkung am Handgelenk. Chirurg 48, 431 (1977).

Perves, J., Rigaud, A., Badelon, L.: Fracture par décapitation du grand os avec déplacement dorsal du corps de l'os simultant une dislocation carpienne. Rev. Orthop. 24, 251 (1937).

Rehbein, F.: Zur Behandlung des veralteten Kahnbeinbruches und der Kahnbeinpseud-arthrose der Hand. Langenbecks Arch. Chir. 260, 356 (1947).

Schmier, A. A., Meyers, M. P.: Bilateral osteochondritis of the pisiform. J. Bone Joint Surg. 21, 789 (1931).

Stack, J. K.: End results of excision of carpal bones. Arch. Surg. 57, 245 (1948).

Stein, F., Siegel, M. W.: Naviculo-capitate fracture syndrome. J. Bone Joint Surg. A 51, 391 (1969).

Steinhäuser, J.: Möglichkeiten und Grenzen der transnaviculo-lunaren Resektionsarthro-plastik der Hand. Handchirurgie 1, 50 (1969).

Verdan, G., Narakas, A.: Fractures and pseudarthrosis of the scaphoid. Surg. Clin. North Am. 48, 1083 (1968).

Wagner, C. J.: Fracture–dislocations of the wrist. Clin. Orthop. 15, 181 (1959).

Weller, S.: Anatomisch-funktionelle Grundlagen der Behandlung von Frakturen der Handwurzelknochen. Hefte Unfallheilkd. 75, 134 (1963).

Wilhelm, A., Sperling, M.: Zur Technik der zentralen Navicularespanung. Chirurg 34, 29 (1963).

Wipfli, W.: Operative Behandlung von Navicularepseudarthrosen der Hand. Zürich: Dis-sertation 1961.

Woiss, C., Laskin, R. S., Spinner, M.: Irreducible transscaphoid perilunar dislocation. J. Bone Joint Surg. A 52, 565 (1970).

Thumb Injuries

The importance of the thumb as the only element that can oppose the long fingers cannot be overemphasized. Of course, the management of thumb injuries basically follows the principles that apply to hand surgery in general. Due to its unique importance in grasping, however, there are several additional principles that pertain mainly to the indications for amputations and reconstructive operations on the thumb.

I. Amputation

1) Amputation is indicated only if all four vessels supplying the thumb are severed. The preservation of a single dorsal vascular bundle is usually sufficient to nourish the thumb.

2) If amputation is unavoidable, the base of the first metacarpal must be preserved if possible owing to its importance in thumb reconstruction.

3) Even the extensive loss of soft tissue is no grounds for amputation. The thumb can be preserved by plastic measures (tubed pedicle, abdominal skin pouch) and its sensation later restored (neurovascular island flaps).

4) In amputating injuries, every millimeter of bone length is valuable. This means that secondary amputation with shortening of the bone is to be avoided. Instead, the bone length should be preserved and the stump covered by plastic means.

In this age of microsurgery, the "reattachment" of a severed portion of the thumb is no longer a matter of pure academic interest. This statement is important in view of the fact that an increasing number of injured persons are bringing traumatically amputated members with them to the hospital.

II. Fractures of the Thumb

Treatment follows the rules of fracture therapy in hand surgery and is generally conservative. In Bennet's fracture–dislocation at the base of the first metacarpal, accurate osteosynthesis to avoid secondary arthrosis is desirable in view of the importance of the saddle joint for thumb motility (Figures 139–141).

III. Thumb Joint Injuries

A. Terminal and Basal Joints

Where these joints are concerned, stability ranks above motility. A strong ulnar ligament at the basal joint is indispensible for grasping. A rupture of this ligament requires operative correction (Figure 118). In the interest of stability and a painless grasp, the indications for arthrodesis are somewhat broader for these two joints.

B. Saddle Joint

As the "key joint" of the thumb, the saddle joint requires motility more than stability. All factors that impair the mobility of this joint—especially injuries that lead to secondary arthrosis and thus to a painful limitation of motion—must be remedied. These measures include:

1) Accurate operative care of Bennet's fracture–dislocation.
2) Operative correction of a post-traumatic recurrent dislocation or subluxation.

In addition to Bunnell's technique of lashing the saddle joint with the fascia or palmar tendon (Figure 172a–c), we presently prefer the author's technique of transferring the short extensor tendon of the thumb, which also restores the necessary stability of the saddle joint without impairing its motility (Figure 173a–c).

If grasping is no longer made painful by secondary arthrosis, the situation can be improved either by arthrodesis in palmar abduction (Figure 174b) or by extirpation of the trapezium (Figure 175). The approach is shown in Figure 172b. Restraint is advised regarding the indication for these operations, which is present only if there is a severe, painful impairment of grasp that is causing the patient distress.

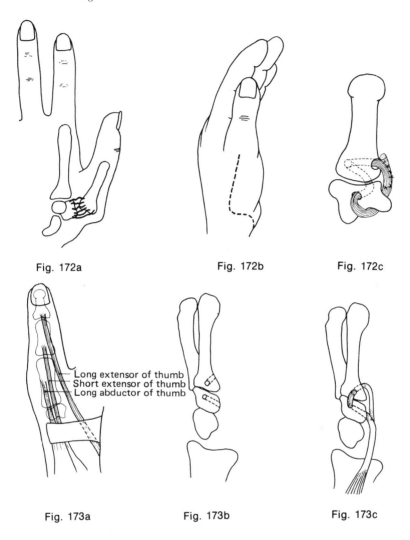

Fig. 172a   Fig. 172b   Fig. 172c

Long extensor of thumb
Short extensor of thumb
Long abductor of thumb

Fig. 173a   Fig. 173b   Fig. 173c

IV. Division of the Long Extensor Tendon of the Thumb

A. Fresh Injury

The central tendon stump generally retracts a considerable distance. An auxiliary incision is a better means of locating the stump than "blind fishing." The tendon is reunited by Lengemann suture. The immobilization and postoperative treatment follow the principles that apply to tendon surgery (Figure 176a,b).

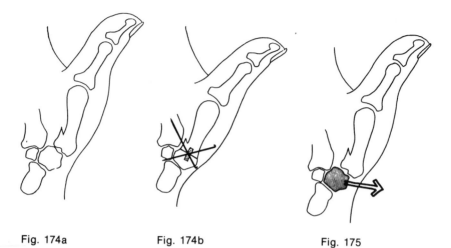

Fig. 174a   Fig. 174b   Fig. 175

B. Old Injury: Untreated Division, "Drummer's Paralysis"
   (Fatigue Rupture)

This functional loss can be corrected by transferring the extensor tendon of the index finger, which is found ulnar to the second common extensor tendon (Figure 177a,b).

V. Division of the Long Flexor Tendon of the Thumb

The first ray also has its "no man's land" (Figure 178, II). However, because only *one* long tendon is found there, the prognosis is better than

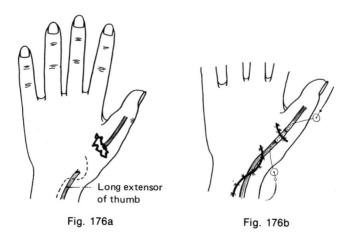

Long extensor
of thumb

Fig. 176a   Fig. 176b

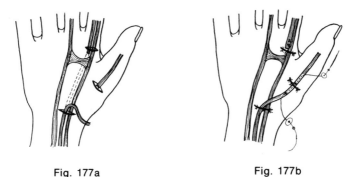

Fig. 177a   Fig. 177b

for the long fingers, even in the case of primary suture by the "suture at a distance" technique. Nevertheless, a flexion contracture sometimes results due to the unavoidable loss of tendon tissue. Therefore a more differentiated procedure is recommended:

A. Injury Distal to "No Man's Land"

The long flexor tendon of the thumb is lengthened in Z-fashion near its origin in the forearm such that the distal end of the central tendon stump can be reinserted into the distal phalanx, while the distal tendon stump is sacrificed (Figure 179).

B. Injury in "No Man's Land"

The free grafting of a palmar tendon according to the rules of flexor tendon surgery is indicated. The operation can also be performed as a primary measure with good results (Figure 180).

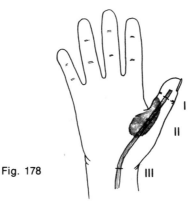

Fig. 178

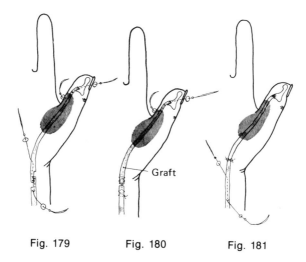

Fig. 179   Fig. 180   Fig. 181

C. Injury Central to "No Man's Land"

Primary suture by the method of Dychno-Bunnell or "suture at a distance" by Lengemann suture (Figure 181) is performed.

VI. Cicatricial Adduction Contracture of the Thumb

The thumb is opposable only if it can be abducted palmarward. Cicatricial contracture of the first interdigital space must therefore be corrected. Z-plasty can be employed in mild cases, otherwise the scar must be interrupted by rotation flaps from the dorsum of the hand (Figure 182a,b).

VII. Thumb Reconstruction

A. Indications

The loss of both phalanges of the thumb is generally no reason in itself to sacrifice a healthy finger to pollicization, especially since metacarpolysis provides a good operative means of at least partially replacing the thumb function if adductability can be preserved (Figure 183a,b). The

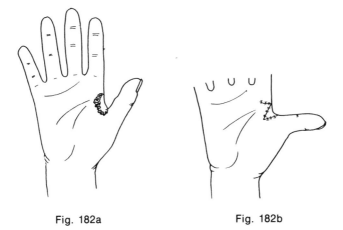

Fig. 182a   Fig. 182b

patient generally adjusts remarkably quickly to the situation and can compensate for the lost thumb by developing substitute forms of grasp.

Reconstruction of the thumb is indicated if most of the first metacarpal is lost, or if the loss of the two phalanges of the thumb is accompanied by the loss or serious injury of long fingers which makes it impossible to execute the power grip.

The patient should be informed of the possibility of thumb reconstruction immediately after the loss of the thumb, but he should not be pressed to undergo the operation, which is best done (if at all) several months after the patient has resumed work. The reason is that, as in all plastic surgery, the patient's expectations far exceed that which can actually be accomplished. However, if he has been at work for 6 months, perhaps his attitude will have changed toward the operation he so desperately wanted at first, and the physician will have time to judge whether the operation is still warranted at all.

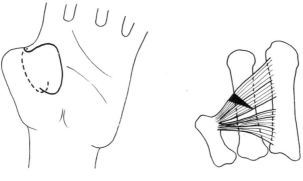

Fig. 183a   Fig. 183b

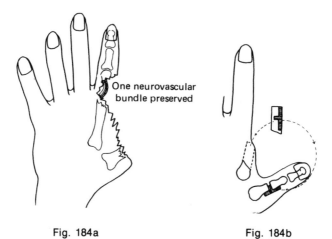

One neurovascular
bundle preserved

Fig. 184a   Fig. 184b

Primary thumb reconstruction may be necessary if, during the course of primary care, a thumb can be formed from a finger or finger remnant that is suitable for that purpose but would otherwise fall victim to amputation (Mittelbach, K. Schmidt, Zrubecky; Figure 184a,b). Because this procedure cannot always be anticipated, it may also have legal consequences if the patient has not given his consent. Schönberger has examined this question in detail within the context of "special circumstances" in his monograph on industrial accidents.

B. Qualities of a Reconstructed Thumb

Hilgenfeldt places the following requirements on the reconstructed thumb:

1) It may be shorter than a natural thumb, but must allow the pinch and power grips to be made.
2) It may be stiff if the saddle joint is mobile.
3) It must have sensation.
4) The patient must be able to move it with sufficient force.
5) It should feel like a thumb to the patient.

C. Techniques of Thumb Reconstruction

1. Pollicization of a Finger (Hilgenfeldt)

In principle, any long finger or long finger remnant with intact volar neurovascular bundles can be used in the construction of a thumb. Even

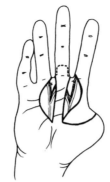

Fig. 185

a single neurovascular bundle on the finger to be pollicized is sufficient for nutrition. The deep flexor tendon of the donor finger should be attached to the stump of the long flexor of the thumb in order to provide correct organic sensation (Figure 185). The lengthening of the first metacarpal by the second metacarpal, with the accompanying loss of the index finger, is based on the same principle (Figure 186a,b).

2. Bone Graft and Tubed Pedicle Flap

A thumb may be constructed by means of a bone graft covered with a tubed pedicle flap and the secondary restoration of sensation by sensory transfer.

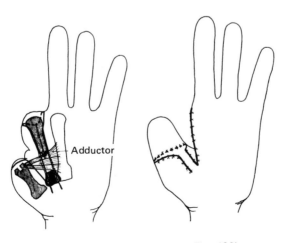

Fig. 186a   Fig. 186b

3. Nicoladoni Thumb

The replacement of the thumb with the big toe is again achieving significance owing to the advanced microsurgical suturing techniques developed in neural and vascular surgery. The restoration of sensation in the graft following microsurgical neuroanastomosis is reported.

4. Additional Techniques

Obviously, the subject of thumb reconstruction cannot be treated exhaustively in such a brief discussion. The interested reader can refer to Hilgenfeldt's monograph, which, though written 30 years ago, is still timely. He will be surprised to learn of the many possibilities that exist for correcting the disorders of grasp caused by finger losses once one is well acquainted with the principles of hand surgery.

Bibliography

Buck-Gramcko, D.: Wiederherstellung der Sensibilität bei Teilverlust des Daumens. Langebecks Arch. Chir. 299, 99 (1961).

Buck-Gramcko, D.: Verlängerung des 1. Mittelhandknochens zur Funktionsverbesserung der Hand bei Verlust des Daumens und mehrerer Langfinger. Monatsschr. Unfallheilkd. 73, 29 (1970).

Chase, R. A.: An alternative to pollicisation in subtotal thumb reconstruction. Plast. Reconstr. Surg. 44, 421 (1969).

Cho, K. O.: Translocation of the abductor pollicis longus tendon. A treatment for chronic subluxation of the thumb carpometacarpal joint. J. Bone Joint Surg. A 52, 1166 (1970).

Eaton, R. G., Littler, J. W.: A study of the basal joint of the thumb. Treatment of its disabilities by fusion. J. Bone Joint Surg. A 51, 661 (1969).

Finseth, F., May, J. W., Smith, R. J.: Composite groin flaps with iliacal-bone flap for primary thumb reconstruction. J. Bone Joint Surg. A 58, 131 (1976).

Flatt, A. E.: An indication for shortening of the thumb. J. Bone Joint Surg. A 46, 1534 (1964).

Fleischer, H.: Die operative Versorgung von Spontanrupturen und Verletzungen der Sehne des langen Daumenstreckers. Monatsschr. Unfallheilkd. 68, 224 (1965).

Freilinger, G.: Zur Autoreplantation des Daumens. Acta Chir. Aust. 2, 88 (1970).

Kelleher, J. G., Sullivan, J. G.: Daumenersatz durch Verlagerung des 5. Fingers (Ref.). Plast. Reconstr. Surg. 21, H. 6 (1958).

Matev, J. B.: Thumb reconstruction after amputation at the metacarpophalangeal joint by bone lengthening. J. Bone Joint Surg. A 52, 957 (1970).

Merle d'Aubigné, R., Lataste, J.: Les arthrodèses du poignet. Rev. Orthop. 42, 185 (1956).

Mittelbach, H. R.: Primärer Daumenersatz. Ein Beitrag zur operativen Daumenbildung. Monatsschr. Unfallheilkd. 64, 102 (1961).

Müller, M.: Der autoplastische Daumenersatz. Praxis 46, 441N (1957).

Nicoladoni, K.: Daumenplastik und organischer Ersatz der Fingerspitze. Arch. Klin. Chir. 27, 606 (1900).

Nicoladoni, K.: Weitere Erfahrungen mit Daumenplastik. Arch Klin. Chir. 69, 695 (1912).

Nigst, H.: Zur Frage der Wiederherstellung der Funktion des M. extensor pollicis brevis nach Spontanrupturen und Verletzungen. Helv. Chir. Acta 22, 504 (1955).

Payr, E.: Daumenersatz durch die Großzehe. Dtsch. Z. Chir. 157, 395 (1918).

Perthes, G.: Plastischer Ersatz des verlorenen Daumens. Münch. Med. Wochenschr. 113 (1919).

Pitzler, K.: Der Daumenersatz aus dem zweiten Mittelhandknochen. Bruns Beitr. Klin. Chir. 217, 321 (1969).

Pohl, J.: Schädigungen der Gelenke des ersten Fingerstrahles und ihre Bedeutung für die Funktion der Hand. Hefte Unfallheilkd. 75, 137 (1963).

Poigenfürst, J.: Die Entfernung des Os multangulum majus bei Arthrose des Sattelgelenkes. Z. Orthop. 95, 212 (1961).

Reid, D. A. C.: Reconstruction of the thumb. J. Bone Joint Surg. B 42, 444 (1960).

Röding, H.: Zur Frage der Verpflanzung der Ext. ind. propr.-Sehne. Monatsschr. Unfallheilkd. 65, 431 (1962).

Schmidt, A., Zrubecky, G.: Wiederherstellung einer Greiffunktion nach vollständigem Verlust der Langfinger und einem Teilverlust des Daumens. Zentralbl. Chir. 85, 2397 (1960).

Schmidt, K.: Primäre Daumenbildung als Beitrag zum operativen Daumenersatz. Zentralbl. Chir. 82, 1627 (1957).

Spinner, M.: Fashioned transpositional flap for soft tissue adduction contracture of the thumb. Plast. Reconstr. Surg. 44, 345 (1969).

Verdan, C.: The reconstruction of the thumb. Surg. Clin. North Am. 48, 1033 (1968).

Wilflingseder, P.: Zum Problem der Daumenautotransplantation. Monatsschr. Unfallheilkd. 71, 68 (1968).

Zrubecky, G.: Zur Wiederherstellung der Sensibilität an der Kuppe eines aus Bauchhaut gebildeten, gefühllosen Daumens. Zentralbl. Chir. 85, 1671 (1960).

Compressive Nerve Injuries of the Hand

Compressive nerve injuries of the upper extremities are commonly found in hand surgery if, when the corresponding subjective complaints are present, the physician thinks of the possibility of neuropathy, obtains an accurate prehistory, and searches for objective neurological symptoms.

For anatomical reasons, the focus of compressive sensory and motor neuropathy in the hand region should not be sought in the hand itself, but at the more centrally located isthmic regions in the course of the nerve. [Exceptions are injuries to the brachial plexus itself (cervical rib, costoclavicular compression, scalenus syndrome) or root lesions associated with vertebral injuries.] Compressive nerve injuries result from a change in the boundaries of the passage traversed by the nerve. This may be due to space-consuming inflammatory and degenerative processes, accessory and atavistic anatomical substrates, motor components, an endocrine-induced increase of tissue turgor, or the results of trauma. The latter may involve malunited fractures, uncorrected (lunate) dislocations, or cicatrization subsequent to a blunt or sharp trauma. For this reason, and because of their considerable significance to social medicine, a special chapter has been devoted to compressive nerve injuries.

I. Localization of the Compression Injury

A. Median Nerve

1) Carpal tunnel.
2) The crossing of the median nerve with the pronator teres muscle:

damage may occur to the nerve trunk in this region, as well as isolated injuries to the volar interosseous nerve.

B. Ulnar Nerve

1) Guyon's canal of the wrist: the nerve trunk or its branches may be
   injured in this region.
2) Ulnar groove at the elbow joint.

C. Radial Nerve

1) Passage of the radial nerve through the supinator muscle (supinator
   syndrome).
2) Hiatus of the radial nerve (midlevel radial paralysis).
3) Proximal head of triceps muscles before the nerve enters the radial
   intermuscular septum (proximal radial compression syndrome).

II. Diagnosis

The diagnosis is based on an accurate anamnesis, a general clinical
and subtle neurological diagnosis, including electromyography if possible, and an x-ray examination.

A. Subjective Complaints

1. Paresthesia

Paresthesia can often be localized in the region supplied by a nerve only
after very intensive questioning and may be limited to the autonomous
zones there.

2. Pain

Pains radiate upward from the forearm to the shoulder and neck region, often worsen at night, and are sometimes confused with cervical
root lesions.

B. Objective Evidence

1. Motor and/or Sensory Losses in the Region
   Supplied by a Nerve

The concurrent involvement of several nerves is possible, especially at the wrist. An attempt must be made to locate the level of the lesion, taking into account the tapping sign (Hofmann) and the localization of pain on stretching. In experienced hands, electromyography is an indispensible tool for objectively locating the level of the lesion.

2. X-ray Examination in the Standard Planes, with
   Additional Central Views (Hart and Gaynor) of the Wrist
   (Figures 152, 153)

These views provide information on bone injuries, malunions, the dislocation of isolated fragments, uncorrected dislocations, and the presence of foreign bodies. All complaints and neurological symptoms may occur together, singly, or in a variety of combinations, as well as in varying intensity. There is often a marked discrepancy between the severity of the subjective sensations and the objective signs, which may be slight.

3. Neurological Examination

The operative treatment of compressive nerve injuries requires an accurate knowledge of neurology and topographic and functional anatomy. Only in this way can the lesions be correctly localized, which is an essential prerequisite for a successful operation. The damage is not always visible macroscopically in the exposed nerve. This makes it all the more important to accurately locate the level of the lesion, a job which should always be done in cooperation with a neurologist.

III. Indications

It should be remembered that the operations necessary to free an entrapped nerve are relatively mild compared with the possible harm done by the uncorrected lesion. Nerve exposure is indicated if the following conditions are present:

1) There are distinct motor and/or sensory losses.

2) The level of the lesion can be accurately determined.
3) No spontaneous remission of the objective losses or subjective complaints has occurred within 8 weeks after the trauma.

IV. Therapy

Conservative treatment with immobilization or antiproliferative medication brings at best only temporary relief in the fully developed compression syndrome. Local injection therapy with cortisone, for example, can even cause additional damage.

The object of the only possible recourse, operative treatment, is the decompression of the nerve. Depending on the localization, the following operations are available individually or in combination:

Enlargement of the nerve passage.
Neurolysis.
Rerouting of the nerve.

If the traumatic origin of the lesion has not been established prior to operation, tissue must be taken from the nerve passage for histological examination in order to facilitate subsequent evaluation for insured patients if need be.

Post-traumatic compressive injuries of the median nerve in the carpal canal, the ulnar nerve in the region of Guyon's canal, and the ulnar groove are by far the most common. We shall thus center our discussion on their operative treatment. *The operative treatment of all other compression syndromes should be left to the experienced surgeon.*

A. Median Nerve

1. Anatomy

The guides at the wrist are the long palmar tendon ventral to the median nerve and the radial flexor tendon of the wrist radial to the nerve. In the carpal canal, bounded at the sides and bottom by the carpal bones and at the top by the transverse carpal ligament, the median nerve follows a course on the finger flexors and divides into its terminal branches while still in the canal or at its distal border.

2. Exposure of the Median Nerve at the Wrist
   and in the Carpal Canal

Exposure is by a zigzag cutaneous incision at the wrist which extends to the thenar crease. If the long palmar is variant, its tendon is sectioned. The transverse carpal ligament is split well into the palm or is sparingly resected. During neurolysis, any scar tissue present is removed. The problem of the extirpation of the lunate bone in the case of old dislocations is mentioned in passing. Special attention should be given the muscular branch for the thenar, which arises at a point that is often located far centrally, as well as the sensory palmar branch, which runs volar to the transverse carpal ligament. The wound is closed by cutaneous suture, *without* suture of the transverse carpal ligament. The incision permits the simultaneous inspection of Guyon's canal (Figure 187).

B. Ulnar Nerve

1. Anatomy

The ulnar nerve is most prone to compressive injury in its course in the ulnar groove on the posterior surface of the medial epicondyle of the humerus and in the course of its deep branch at the wrist in Guyon's canal. Protected by the ulnar head of the triceps, the ulnar nerve enters the easily palpable groove behind the ulnar epicondyle at a point dorsal

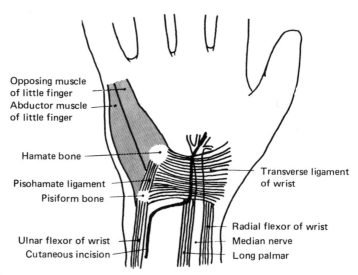

Fig. 187

to the ulnar intermuscular septum; there it lies adjacent to the bone without padding, covered only by a layer of connective tissue and perhaps a ligament or epitrochleoanconeus muscle. In a distal direction it disappears below the tendinous arch of the ulnar flexor muscle of the wrist between the two heads of this muscle, whereupon it gives off the first muscular branch to supply the wrist flexors.

At the wrist the nerve follows its guide muscle, the ulnar flexor of the wrist, to Guyon's canal, bounded on the sides by the hamate and pisiform and at the bottom by the transverse carpal ligament, and roofed by the volar carpal ligament and offshoots from the dorsal carpal ligament. In this very superficial canal, the nerve divides into a superficial sensory branch to the fourth and fifth fingers, and a deep motor branch, which divides deep in the canal to supply the hypothenar and the small hand muscles (interosseous muscles and adductor muscle of the thumb).

2. Exposure of the Ulnar Nerve at the Wrist and in Guyon's Canal

A zigzag incision is made at the wrist. The ulnar nerve is located by its guide muscle, the ulnar flexor of the wrist, and followed distally into the hypothenar. The roof of Guyon's canal is split or sparingly resected to expose the individual branches. Scar tissue or bony ridges following fractures are removed. The superficial portions of the ligaments are not sutured, only the skin (Figure 188).

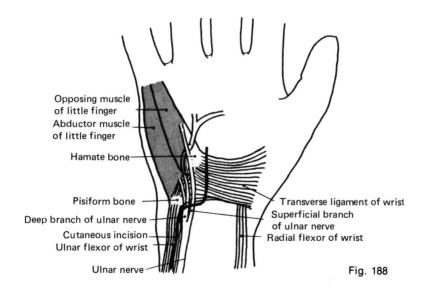

Opposing muscle of little finger
Abductor muscle of little finger
Hamate bone
Pisiform bone
Deep branch of ulnar nerve
Cutaneous incision
Ulnar flexor of wrist
Ulnar nerve
Transverse ligament of wrist
Superficial branch of ulnar nerve
Radial flexor of wrist

Fig. 188

3. Exposure of the Ulnar Nerve at the Elbow Joint

A curved longitudinal incision is made corresponding to the ulnar groove in the epicondyle line. The connective tissue roof of the ulnar groove, often altered by scarring, is split from the emergence of the nerve from the triceps muscle to its first branch points after its entry into the ulnar flexor muscle of the wrist. The tendinous arch of the ulnar flexor of the wrist is sectioned. Neurolysis is continued up to the point where the first muscular branch arises. Watch for the presence of a ligament or epitrochleoanconeus muscle. The ligament must be sectioned, while the muscle is severed at its insertion and reinserted after the nerve is freed. If possible, and especially after fractures with cubitus valgus or in the presence of a dislocation or subluxation of the nerve or an atavistic muscle, the nerve is rerouted beneath the subcutaneous fatty tissue on the ventral side (Figure 189).

V. Postoperative Care

The pain and paresthesia usually disappear shortly after surgery, often abruptly. The time and extent of the return of lost sensory and motor functions are dependent on the extent and duration of the nerve damage. Even more important is a sufficiently long (several months if necessary) and consistent program of electrotherapy in conjunction with exercise under the direction of a physiotherapist. The latter treatment is often amazingly effective in evoking compensatory mechanisms for

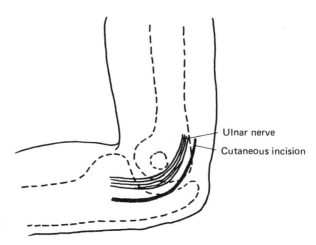

Ulnar nerve

Cutaneous incision

Fig. 189

motor and sensory losses. If important functions remain impaired for more than 1 year, the possibility of a transfer operation must be considered.

Bibliography

Barthold, G.: Die handchirurgische Bedeutung und Diagnostik des ulnaren Canalis carpi. Zentralbl. Chir. 85, 606 (1960).

Brooks, D. M.: Traumatic ulnar neuritis. J. Bone Joint Surg. B 32, 291 (1950).

Brooks, D. M.: Nerve compression syndromes. J. Bone Joint Surg. B 45, 445 (1963).

Cameron, B. M.: Occlusion of the ulnar artery with impending gangrene of the fingers relieved by section of the volar carpal ligament. J. Bone Joint Surg. A 36, 406 (1954).

Cannon, B. W., Love, J.: Tardy median palsy: median thenar neuritis amentable to surgery. Surgery 20, 210 (1946).

Conway, F. M.: Traumatic ulnar neuritis with especial reference to the late or tardy ulnar paralysis. Ann. Surg. 425 (1933).

Cypener, N.: Posterior interosseus nerve lesions. J. Bone Joint Surg. B 46, 361 (1964).

Dupont, C., Cloutier, G. E., Prévost, Y., Dion, M. A.: Ulnar-tunnel syndrome at the wrist. J. Bone Joint Surg. A 47, 757 (1965).

Guyon, F.: Note sur une disposition anatomique propre á la face anterieure de la région du poignet et non encore décrite par le docteur. Bull. Soc. Anat. Paris 6, 184 (1861).

Hart, V. L., Gaynor, V.: Roentgenographic study of the carpal canal. J. Bone Joint Surg. 23, 382 (1941).

Howard, F. M.: Ulnar nerve palsy in wrist fracture. J. Bone Joint Surg. A 43, 1197 (1961).

Moffat, J. A.: Traumatic neuritis of the deep palmar branch of the ulnar nerve. Can. Med. Assoc. J. 91, 230 (1964).

Rosen, S. v.: Ein Fall von Thrombose in der Arteria ulnaris nach Einwirkung von stumpfer Gewalt. Acta Chir. Scand. 73, 500 (1934).

Sharrard, W. J. W.: Anterior interosseus neuritis. J. Bone Joint Surg. B 50, 804 (1968).

Spinner, M.: The arcade of Frohse and its relationship to posterior interosseus nerve paralysis. J. Bone Joint Surg. B 50, 809 (1968).

Teece, L. G.: Thrombosis of the ulnar artery. Aust. N. Z. J. Surg. 19, 156 (1949).

Wilhelm, A.: Neues über Druckschäden des N. ulnaris und N. radialis. Handchirurgie 2, 143 (1970).

Transfer Operations for Irreparable Nerve Damage

These operations are an exercise from the "high school" of hand surgery and are most definitely not for the beginner! Even the inexperienced surgeon, however, must know at least the indications and contraindications for the major transfers, as well as their possibilities and limits so that he can properly guide and advise his patients. Experience has taught that even in peacetime and despite the new microsurgical techniques developed for the suturing and grafting of nerves, transfers have remained an important technique for dealing with irreparable nerve damage. Unfortunately, corrective operations are frequently overlooked due to physician ignorance or are rejected by the patient because of poor psychological guidance.

I. General Indications

Generally speaking, a transfer is indicated only if nerve damage cannot be compensated for by training, there are no prospects for spontaneous regeneration, and all possibilities for restoring the continuity of the nerve have been exhausted. The indication for the transfer and the timing of the operation (generally about 1 year after the injury) should be determined in close cooperation with the neurologist, who must give the surgeon accurate documentation not only on muscular losses, but also on the intact innervation of the muscles selected for the transfer.

A. Special Indications for Relatively Simple Motor Transfers

1. Drop Hand in High Radial Paralysis

The wrist cannot be actively raised from its flexed position. Extension of the thumb and the basal joints of the long fingers is impossible, and the thumb cannot be abducted. The loss of all extensors has led to an active insufficiency of the flexors and thus to a weak closure of the fist.

2. Oath Hand in High Median Paralysis

This results from the loss of the three deep radial flexors (long flexor of the thumb and deep flexors of the second and third fingers), all four superficial finger flexors, and the opposing muscle.

3. Loss of Thumb Opposition in Peripheral Median Paralysis

4. Claw Hand in Peripheral Ulnar Paralysis

The loss of all intrinsic muscles, including the adductor of the thumb, leads to the disturbance of muscle balance (intrinsic muscles flex the basal joints but extend the middle and terminal joints) and thus to a marked extension of the basal joints, flexion of the middle and terminal joints, and loss of the power grip. The pinch grip is also weakened by the loss of abduction of the index finger (first interosseous).

5. Claw Hand in Combined Peripheral Ulnar–Median Paralysis

The additional loss of thumb opposition leads virtually to the complete functional disability of the hand.

Important differential diagnosis: ischemic contracture (usually following supracondylar humerus fracture during childhood).

B. Special Indications for Sensory Transfers

1) Complete loss of sensation in the region supplied by the median nerve, and in rare cases the ulnar nerve (here only within the context of the operative construction of secondary forms of grasp).
2) Restoration of sensation in functionally critical zones in the region of grafts: caution is advised, for neurovascular island flaps do not develop a new organic sensation.

II. Contraindications

1) Patient over 45–50 years of age.
2) Patient lacks the will to cooperate and lacks intelligence (no desire to work, pension seekers, neurotics).
3) Absence of protective sensation.
4) Poor trophicity.
5) Poor scar conditions.
6) Arthrogenic contractures.

Only contraindications 5 and 6 can be eliminated by preliminary surgical measures.

III. Techniques

A. Motor Losses

In view of the variety of motor transfer techniques known, it is impossible to discuss them in detail. All the techniques, however, are based on the same principle: by the transposition (transinsertion) of dispensible innervated tendons to a paralyzed kinetic chain, an attempt is made to compensate for the functional loss by imitating as closely as possible the natural lines of pull. This procedure is combined with the tenodesis and arthrodesis of second-order joints if necessary in order to release tendons for the restoration of important functions. Numerous atypical situations may compel the surgeon to develop combinative skills of his own. In general, the following techniques have proved valuable for major motor nerve losses:

1. High Radial Paralysis

This can be corrected by use of double-tendon transfers: ulnar flexor of the wrist into common extensor of the fingers and long extensor of the thumb, and radial flexor of the wrist into long abductor and short extensor of the thumb. The tenodesis or even arthrodesis of the wrist may be desirable under certain conditions (Bauer, Franke, Perthes; Figure 190).

2. High Median Paralysis

The short radial extensor of the wrist serves as the motor for the long flexor of the thumb, the fourth superficial flexor is used to produce op-

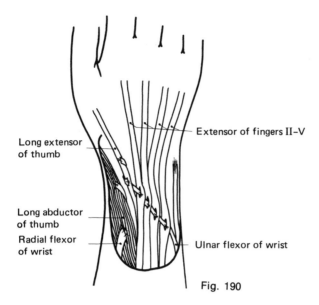

Long extensor
of thumb

Extensor of fingers II–V

Long abductor
of thumb

Radial flexor
of wrist

Ulnar flexor of wrist

Fig. 190

position, and the deep flexor tendons of the second and third fingers are attached to the ulnar-supplied fourth and fifth deep flexors, whose force can be increased by the brachioradialis (Brand, Bunnell, Riordan, Thompson, Figure 191; opposition transfer, Figure 192).

3. Loss of Opposition of the Thumb
   (Peripheral Median Paralysis)

The fourth superficial flexor used as the motor is the simplest technique (Thompson; Figure 192).

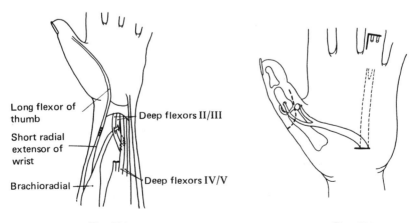

Long flexor of
thumb

Deep flexors II/III

Short radial
extensor of
wrist

Brachioradial

Deep flexors IV/V

Fig. 191

Fig. 192

4. Peripheral Ulnar Paralysis

In this form of paralysis it is most important that hyperextension of the basal joints of the long fingers be corrected in order to restore muscle balance and thus the action of the finger flexors. The simplest and surest approach is Zancolli's proximal advancement of the capsule with its tenodesis effect (Figure 193a,b). Bunnell's suggestion for transferring superficial tendons to the dorsal aponeurosis has proved to be less certain and often acts only by virtue of its tenodesis effect. To stabilize the pinch grip, abduction of the index finger is restored with the tendon of the extensor of the index finger, and the basal joint of the thumb is stabilized by arthrodesis (Littler).

5. Combined Peripheral Median–Ulnar Paralysis

In this case Zancolli's operation to correct hyperextension of the basal long finger joints is combined with opposition transfer.

B. Sensory Losses

A motor transfer is still worthwhile even if the volar surface has only protective sensation. Tactile gnosis is better, however, at least in the median-innervated region. The prehensile hand remnant left after multiple finger losses is worth little without sensation, an insensible thumb is almost useless, and even the loss of sensation in only certain fingers may make it impossible for the patient to practice his normal profession. This situation can be improved by various modifications of the sensory transfer operation:

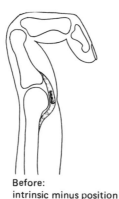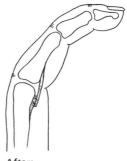

Before:
intrinsic minus position

After:
intrinsic plus position

Fig. 193a   Fig. 193b

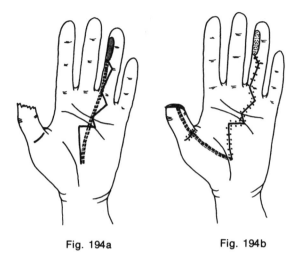

Fig. 194a   Fig. 194b

1) Neurovascular island flaps (Littler, Zrubecky; Figure 194a,b).
2) Dorsoradial flaps from the index ray (Hilgenfeldt; Figure 195a,b).
3) Any other local pedicle flaps capable of restoring cutaneous sensation.

IV. Limits

Before the operation the patient naturally envisions a more or less complete restoration of lost functions. The physician must therefore tell

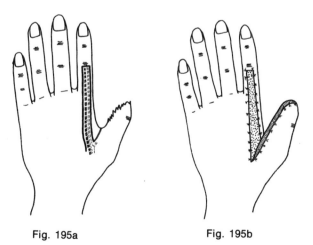

Fig. 195a   Fig. 195b

the patient beforehand that transfer operations can never fully compensate for the loss of a natural function, largely because the original functions of the motors (which may be termed "second-degree functions") must be relinquished. In paralysis of the intrinsic muscles, moreover, reconstructive operations cannot replace their proprioceptive functions.

Nevertheless, even a modest substitute function is better than no function at all, if only to meet the most basic needs of everyday life.

Bibliography

Bauer, K. H.: Wesentliche Vereinfachung der Radialisplastik. Chirurg 17–18, 1 (1947).

Bauer, K. H.: Weitere Vereinfachung der Perthesplastik für Radialislähmung. Chirurg 17–18, 501 (1947).

Böhler, J.: Lähmung der Binnenmuskeln der Hand, Ersatzoperation mit Superficialisverlagerung und Opponensplastik. Langenbecks Arch. Chir. 299, 140 (1961).

Brand, P. W.: Paralytic claw hand. With special reference to paralysis in leprosy and treatment by the sublimis transfer of *Stiles* and *Bunnell.* J. Bone Joint Surg. B 40, 618 (1958).

Brown, P. W.: Zancolli capsulorrhaphy for ulnar claw hand. J. Bone Joint Surg. A 52, 868 (1970).

Bunnell, St.: Tendon transfers in the hand and forearm. American Academy of Orthopaedic Surgeons Instructional Course Lectures, Vol. VI. Ann Arbor: Edwards 1949.

Cotta, H.: Die Ersatzoperationen bei irreparablen Lähmungen peripherer Nerven Hefte Unfallheilkd. 81, 279 (1965).

Granberry, W. M., Lipscomb, P. R.: Tendon transfers to the hand in brachial palsy. Am. J. Surg. 108, 840 (1964).

Henderson, E. D.: Transfer of wrist extensors and brachioradialis to restore opposition of the thumb. J. Bone Joint Surg. A 44, 513 (1962).

Jacobs, B. J., Thompson, T. C.: Opposition of the thumb and its restoration. J. Bone Joint Surg. A 42, 1039 (1960).

Littler, J. W.: Tendon transfers and arthrodesis in combined median and ulnar nerve paralysis. J. Bone Joint Surg. A 31, 225 (1949).

Littler, J. W.: Neurovascular skin island transfer in reconstructive hand surgery. J. Bone Joint Surg. A 38, 817 (1956).

Omer, G. E., et al.: Neurovascular cutaneous island pedicles for deficient median-nerve sensibility. J. Bone Joint Surg. A 52, 1181 (1970).

Perthes, G.: Über Sehnenoperationen bei irreparabler Radialislähmung. Bruns Beitr. Klin. Chir. 113, 289 (1918).

Riordan, D. C.: Surgery of the paralytic hand. American Academy of Orthopaedic Surgeons Instructional Course Letters, Vol. XVI. St. Louis: Mosby 1959.

Schink, W.: Wiederherstellungschirurgie bei Nervenverletzungen im Bereich der Hand. Hefte Unfallheilkd. 81, 274 (1965).

Schock, J.: Zur Wahl der Ersatzplastik nach irreversibler Radialislähmung. Arch. Orthop. Unfallchir. 49, 663 (1958).

Thompson, T. C.: A modified operation for opponens paralysis. J. Bone Joint Surg. 24, 632 (1942).

Tubiana, R.: Anatomic and physiologic basis for the surgical treatment of paralyses of the hand. J. Bone Joint Surg. A 52, 643 (1969).

Tubiana, R., Dupac, J., Moreau, C.: Restauration de la sensibilité au niveau de la main par transfer d'une transplant cutané hétérodigital muni de son pédicule vasculonerveux. Rev. Chir. Orthop. 46, 163 (1960).

Uriburu, J. J. F., Morchio, F. J., Marin, J. C.: Compression syndrome of the deep motor branch of the ulnar nerve (piso-hamate hiatus syndrome). J. Bone Joint Surg. A 58, 145 (1976).

Witt, A. N.: Die Wiederherstellungsoperationen bei irreparablen Nervenlähmungen der oberen Extremität. Langenbecks Arch. Chir. 301, 942 (1962).

Zrubecky, G.: Ersatzoperationen bei schweren Handverletzungen. Hefte Unfallheilkd. 75, 143 (1963).

Severe Crush Injuries of the Hand

A distinction must be made between open crush injuries with the destruction of skin, bone, tendons, and nerves and closed crush injuries, since the two types of injury require largely different treatment measures. Both injuries are characterized by massive post-traumatic edema, which requires special attention.

I. Severe Open Crush Injury

The care of this injury follows the same principles that apply to severe combined injuries.

A. Immediate Care

It is essential that the following measures be taken:

The skin cover is restored.
The skeleton is repaired by osteosynthesis.
Measures are taken against post-traumatic edema.

It may be extremely difficult to distinguish devitalized soft tissue from viable tissue, even by the "vital coloration" method, and management according to the "emergency with delayed operation" procedure may be warranted. The viability of skin stripped from the hand in degloving injuries is often surprising. Primary plastic replacement of the skin is almost always necessary, however. Secondary skin necrosis is not uncommon and requires prompt necrotomy and plastic repair.

Damaged muscle tissue cannot be sutured. Any attempt to do so will only endanger remaining muscle tissue, because *muscle is not a suturable tissue*. Crush injuries differ from sharp divisions in that in the former injuries, the union of fasciae still present in the hand entails the danger of ischemic necrosis.

The immediate reconstruction of the skeletal formation avoids not only pressure necrosis of the skin through malunions, but also a persistent disturbance of the muscle balance, which may later require tedious reconstructive surgery. The more stable the osteosynthesis, the better the prognosis for hand function, which depends in large measure on an early program of therapeutic exercise because the gliding surfaces of the tendons are always affected even though the continuity of the tendons themselves is often preserved.

A hematoma in the wrist region calls for primary decompression of the carpal canal and the canal of Guyon with a search for fractures of the pisiform and hamulus of the hamate (which may escape x-ray diagnosis) either during the course of primary care or secondarily at the first signs of a nerve compression syndrome.

The measures against post-traumatic edema merit particular attention. Edema is usually less the result of a disturbance of blood flow through the hand than an impairment of the microcirculation combined with the release of vasodilating substances such as histamine and kinins, which also increase the vascular permeability. Vascular dilatations evoked by the pain receptors also play a role.

A certain polypharmacy is necessary to control these factors. This therapy, which is best initiated before the operation, must include the following:

1) Pain relief and autonomic block with maintenance of circulatory regulating mechanisms by lytic cocktail: pethidine–promethazine–Hydergine (0.1 mg dihydroergocornine methansulfonate, 0.1 mg dihydroergocristine methansulfonate and 0.1 mg dihydrocryptine methansulfonate).
2) Medicinal treatment of edema and edema mobilization with osmotically active substances such as diuretics.
3) Antiphlogistic measures (e.g., oxyphenbutazone).
4) Blockage of kinins and maintenance of microcirculation with aprotinin and low molecular weight dextrans.

After the operation the hand is elevated in the position of function. All unimmobilized joints are actively moved through their full range of motion hourly under professional supervision. Pain-relieving medication is given if necessary.

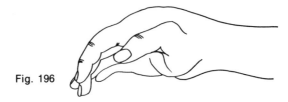

Fig. 196

B. Reconstructive Measures

The care of tendon and nerve injuries is best left to a second operation. This secondary operation must generally be preceded by a period of conservative exercise therapy with the object of preserving or restoring passive joint mobility. In cases of finger loss, the construction of secondary forms of grasp must be considered.

II. Severe Closed Crush Injury

The injury is followed by a rapid, often extreme swelling of the hand, which Rahmel has given the appropriate name of "paw hand" (cheiromegaly) (Figure 196). In this form of edema there is a considerable danger of bursting of the integument due to the skin's low stretch reserves, even if the angiogram shows good perfusion. The immediate and long-term treatment of this injury follows the same principles that apply to edema in open crush injuries:

1) Pain relief and autonomic blockade.
2) Edema treatment and mobilization.
3) Antiphlogistic measures.
4) Blockage of kinins and maintenance of microcirculation.

The decompression of the carpal canal proposed by Rahmel in 1968, with the concurrent decompression of Guyon's canal, has been the primary measure of choice in our clinic for some years.

Bibliography

Koch, S. L.: Crushing injuries of the hand. Surg. Gynecol. Obstet. 114, 629 (1962).
Nicolle, F. W., Chio, B., Woolhouse, F. M.: Restoration of sensory function in severe degloving injuries of the hand. J. Bone Joint Surg. A 48, 1511 (1966).
Rahmel, R.: Das schwere Quetschtrauma der Hand. Chir. Plast. Reconstr. 6, 37 (1969).

Foreign Bodies in the Hand

I. Diagnosis

The diagnosis is based on the anamnesis, the clinical evidence, and the x-ray examination. The latter is effective in revealing metallic bodies, and even objects of low radiopacity can often be visualized by "soft films." It is good practice to mark possible entry wounds with lead pellets. Foreign bodies should always be suspected in infections of uncertain origin, even if no entry wound is immediately evident. This must be borne in mind at operation (see chapter on Hand Infections).

II. Indications and Contraindications to the Operative Removal of Foreign Bodies

The presence of any foreign body in the hand poses the danger of infection, which may not become manifest for days or even weeks. The indication for operative removal is thus present if any of the following conditions are met:

1) The foreign body is visible or palpable.
2) The foreign body has been localized by x-ray.
3) Infection is present.

The indications are limited by the smallness of the foreign body, as in the case of the minute metallic particles sometimes left behind by hammer blows or pinpricks. They are often so tiny that they are not found at operation despite localization by x-ray. Active measures do more harm than good in such cases, especially since these wounds generally heal with no signs of irritation, as demonstrated by the experience of two world wars. If the diagnosis is uncertain, a "wait and see" approach is better than active intervention. As in other operations on the hand, there must be a reasonable relation of risk to gain.

III. Therapy

All operations for the removal of foreign bodies are performed under operating room conditions in a bloodless field. Adequate anesthesia is essential. The incisions must follow the rules that normally apply to hand surgery. Even if it has been localized by x-ray, a small foreign body may be extremely difficult to find at operation. Adequate access must therefore be provided, even if the site of the object is fixed by cannulae inserted in two planes. An electronic image–intensifier makes the job easier. Important anatomical structures must be carefully preserved. Tetanus prophylaxis is advised even in trivial injuries.

A. Foreign Bodies without Manifest Infection

1) Visible foreign bodies sticking into the skin surface are extracted. Excision is unnecessary after disinfection, and the wound is left open.

2) If the foreign body has penetrated to the subcutaneous tissue or farther, the entry wound, track, and bed are excised. The wound may be closed by a few temporary sutures. Delayed primary suture is preferred.

3) If the foreign body has penetrated to the vicinity of important anatomical structures (vessels, nerves, tendons), excision is impossible without risking unnecessary secondary injuries, and immediate wound closure by suture is forbidden. The problem is easily solved, however, by a delayed primary suture.

B. Infected Foreign Bodies

In these cases the rules of septic hand surgery apply (see chapter on Infections of the Hand):

1) Adequate access is attained according to the rules of hand surgery.
2) The foreign body and all necrotic tissue are removed.
3) The wound is left open until the infection is safely under control.

C. Special Foreign Body Injuries

In examining three special types of injury, we shall explain the corresponding treatment procedures, which differ in some respects from the guidelines given above, and thus illustrate principles that can be applied in similar situations.

1. Mercury

Thermometer injuries are relatively common in such places as hospitals and industrial laboratories. The primary removal of the mercury, which is present in the tissue in the form of minute particles, is impossible without the danger of secondary injury. Before long the mercury will become encapsulated in foreign body granulomas. Sooner or later, and before general toxic reactions appear, there will be a painful inflammation followed by liquefaction. We can thus draw the following therapeutic conclusions:

a. *Closure of Wound*
The entry site, usually an incised wound, is excised according to surgical rules and is closed by suture.

b. *Treatment of Granuloma*
If the development of the anticipated granuloma has progressed to a sufficient degree, the hand area is opened according to surgical principles. The mercury can then be removed surgically along with the granuloma. The greatest problem is the timing of the operation. It must be performed after encapsulation has occurred (i.e., the granuloma is visible or palpable), but before progressive inflammatory phenomena or purulent liquefaction have taken place.

2. Spray Guns

Here the foreign material (grease, paint, sand) is blasted into the tissue under high pressure, where it is finely dispersed. The entry wound is extremely small compared with the volume of tissue occupied by the foreign matter. The quantity of material introduced and the depth reached in the tissue vary with the pressure of the spray. The progress of the injury is characterized by four stages:

a. *Initial Stage*
The injury is typically nonpainful and, despite a certain limitation of motion, may be dismissed as trivial.

b. Ischemic Stage

It is not uncommon for large amounts of foreign material to be introduced. The result is a strangulation of the blood flow due to the low stretch reserves of the skin. Clinically, there is a blanching of the affected area, which may be followed by gangrene within a few days.

c. Acute Inflammatory Stage

If the tissue survives the ischemic stage, it is again threatened with gangrene with the onset of the acute inflammatory stage, since the inflammatory exudate taxes the skin's stretch reserves to the utmost.

d. Chronic Inflammatory Stage

The foreign material induces a foreign body reaction that may lead to the loss of function of the affected parts of the extremity and thus to amputation.

We thus have the following requirements in terms of therapy:

Spray-gun injuries must be taken seriously, and stationary treatment is advised. Operative intervention should begin during the ischemic stage. Excision of only the entry wound is insufficient. The affected area must be decompressed by broad exposure according to the rules of hand surgery. The operation is performed in a bloodless field (upper arm tourniquet) under adequate anesthesia. The foreign material is removed to the fullest extent possible. The tendon sheaths are inspected. Imbibed tissue must be sacrificed.

Any residual foreign material is removed surgically during the chronic inflammatory stage.

Sometimes it is impossible to preserve a functional member due to the severity of the injury. This means that a finger may have to be amputated in order to prevent more extensive functional impairment due to stiffening.

---

3. Indelible Pencil

Indelible pencil lead contains an aniline dye that goes into solution in the tissues, leads to edema, necrosis, and liquefaction, and may induce general toxic reactions. The following measures are taken to treat such a wound:

Removal of the lead fragment.
Excision of the entry track.
Removal of all dye-imbibed tissue.
Excision of even simple tracks containing no foreign material.

Whether the wound is subject to primary closure depends on the situation and the time at which treatment is commenced. In case of doubt, a delayed primary suture is always correct.

Bibliography

Brunner, U., Egloff, B.: Handverletzungen mit Spritzpistole. Schweiz. Med. Wochenschr. 96, 1087 (1966).

Rains, A. J. H.: Grease-gun injury to the hand—value of early treatment. Br. Med. J. 1, 626 (1958).

Stark, H. H., Wilson, J. N., Boyes, J. H.: Grease-gun injuries to the hand. J. Bone Joint Surg. A 43, 485 (1961).

Tempest, M. N.: Grease-gun injuries. University Leeds Med. J. 2, 125 (1953).

Infections of the Hand

"Ubi pus, ibi evacua."

This statement remains as true as ever and is a valid rule in septic hand surgery. This fact is unchanged by chemotherapeutics and antibiotics. Surgical therapy must be administered reasonably and sensibly, of course, lest the end result of the "treatment" be a functionally disabled or useless hand. The course of the therapy is largely dictated by the first attending physician. He must distinguish between a pyogenic infection and a primary phlegmonous infection. He must compare and contrast clinical evidence to arrive at a differential diagnosis.

I. Pyogenic Infection

It is usually caused by *Staphylococcus aureus,* leads to early liquefaction, forms an abscess, spreads to adjacent anatomical structures with progressive necrosis, and therefore requires prompt surgical (i.e., operative) treatment. This description includes all pyogenic infections in the volar region of the hand: panaritia, callus abscesses, and suppuration in the fascial spaces of the palm and forearm, as well as furuncles in hair-bearing areas of the hand.

The archaic collective term "panaritium" could be dispensed with, since all the disease pictures that it encompasses can be unambiguously described in terms of other conventional disease names. However, the term has come into such wide usage even among laymen that it will be used here.

A. Diagnosis

Diagnosis is relatively simple if a skin lesion is evident or if the infection has been preceded by a hand operation. In many cases, however, the skin lesion is no longer visible. It is then necessary to question the patient about recent injuries, even trivial ones (e.g., pinpricks), in order to arrive at a correct diagnosis. More certain indications are reports of throbbing and spontaneous pains that worsen at night. Clinically, the inflamed region is characterized by Galen's five signs of inflammation: swelling (tumor), pain (dolor), heat (calor), redness (rubor), and loss of function (functio laesa).

Extreme circumscribed tenderness, even under very slight pressure, marks the site of the pus cavity. The functional impairment resulting from pain and swelling gives an indication of the extent to which the infection has spread. The ordinary pathways by which the infection spreads, especially the tendon sheaths and fascial spaces, must therefore be known (Figure 197a,b). X-ray examination can be used to exclude bone involvement.

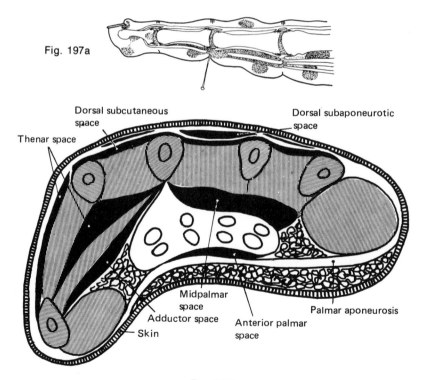

Fig. 197a

Fig. 197b

B. Treatment

1. General Therapy

a. Bandages

So-called traction ointment bandages are the poorest treatment for a pyogenic hand infection, especially if black Ichthyol is used, since it also masks the inflammatory redness!

b. Liquefaction

If the focus of the inflammation can be located, there is no reason to wait until liquefaction has occurred (i.e., until the panaritium has "ripened"), since it is impossible to predict whether the process will progress outward or spread to deeper lying regions (a tendon sheath or joint).

c. Operative Plan

The first operation must be sufficient and therefore the last! The procedure includes not only the drainage of the pus cavity, but also the careful excision of all necrotic tissue. The operation must be carefully planned. An "emergency operation" does more harm than the infection itself.

d. Bacteriological Analysis

A bacteriological analysis of the operative material to determine the resistance of the pathogens is recommended.

e. Incision

Even in septic processes, the incisions must follow the usual rules of hand surgery (i.e., must not cross flexion creases at right angles and should follow skin cleavage lines) (Figure 198). An exception is an outward perforation that has formed or is incipient.

f. Drainage

The wound should be kept open to permit the free drainage of secretions. Klapp's counterincisions are usually unnecessary to promote drainage. The excision of an oval piece of skin prevents the undesired premature cohesion of the wound edges and can thus make drainage unnecessary. It should be remembered that *the success of the treatment depends not on drainage, but on the complete excision of all necrotic tissue!*

Drainage is aided by a layer of ointment gauze or a thin rubber strip if necessary. For deep structures such as tendon sheaths and the wrist, through drainage with plastic catheters is better than any other drainage method.

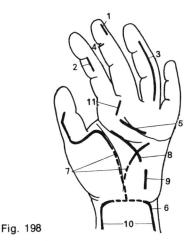

Fig. 198

Tampons should not be used!

Tamponing is unsuitable if septic processes are present. By definition, the loose application of a gauze strip is not tamponing, which is suitable only in cases of diffuse microhemorrhage!

g. Anesthesia

Proper evidence of the seat of the infection requires a steady operating area. Local anesthesia near the seat of the infection raises the danger of bacterial contamination. General anesthesia is best, but plexus anesthesia and subaxillary block anesthesia are acceptable.

h. Tourniquet

Proper evidence of the seat of the infection requires good visibility in the operating field. Only in this way can the iatrogenic injury of functionally important anatomical substrates be avoided. A bloodless field must be produced by means of an upper arm tourniquet. An Esmarch bandage is contraindicated, as it may press pathogenic organisms into the lymph and blood stream. The application of occlusive rubber tubes to the proximal phalanx may lead to fingertip necrosis.

i. Granulating and Extensive Wounds

Granulating surfaces must also be avoided in septic hand surgery. Granulating wounds should therefore be closed by plastic means soon after the infection has subsided. Reverdin grafts are particularly suited for this purpose.

If the incisions are extensive, especially on the forearm, temporary sutures may be applied as a prelude to delayed primary suture after the pus and necrotic tissues have been removed. The edges of the wound are approximated by this method after 48 hours, but not fully adapted.

j. Immobilization

Absolute immobilization of the affected parts in plaster promotes healing, as does elevation for the first 48 hours. The finger joints and the wrist must be immobilized in the position of function. Unaffected fingers remain free. After 2 days, the patient is encouraged to actively exercise all unimmobilized joints, including the shoulder joint.

k. Bandage Change

Avoid superinfection during bandage changes!

l. Postoperative Pain

The absence of pain immediately after the operation confirms the success of the operative treatment of the pyogenic infection. Persisting or recurring pain indicates a progression of the process and requires a second operation. Stationary treatment is indicated at this time.

A persistent infection is sometimes due to the presence of overlooked foreign bodies in the hand. These objects are not glaringly obvious and must be looked for during the secondary operation at the latest.

2. Should Antibiotics Be Given for Pyogenic Infection?

Antibiotics administered enterally or parenterally in the proper dosage can help localize the pyogenic infection and check its further spread, but they can also obscure the disease picture. *To rely entirely on the action of antibiotics is to needlessly jeopardize the function of the hand.*

We recommend the following indications for the use of antibiotics:

1) Panaritium of tendon sheaths, joints, or bones in combination with operative measures.
2) Progression of the inflammatory process after operative treatment in combination with secondary operation.
3) Ascending lymphangitis and lymphadenitis.
4) Sepsis.

In the great majority of cases, pyogenic infections of the hand are caused by gram-positive bacteria, especially *Staphylococcus*. Resistance will probably be present, although it will vary locally. Maximum doses of synthetic penicillins or erythromycin are always correct until the bacterial resistance has been ascertained.

The local application of antibiotics is advised only in the treatment of tendon sheath infections by through drainage. The local application of antibiotics in powdered form is obsolete.

3. X-ray Treatment of Inflammation—Yes or No?

Kühn and Schink et al. advocate radiation therapy as an adjunct to surgical measures, while Edshage rejects it. If the correct operative indication is present, and if the operation is carefully planned and just as carefully performed, this form of therapy is not needed.

4. Hand Baths—Yes or No?

Hand baths generally do more harm than good because they promote the spread of the infection through maceration of the skin. However, they do have their place within the context of postoperative care during bandage changes as a short-term cleansing bath. This bath, incidentally, is less for cleaning the infection wound than its surroundings, which must be cleansed of blood and secretion residue.

5. Special Treatment of Pyogenic Infections

a. *Wound Infections following Hand Operations*
The immediate removal of some or all of the skin sutures with broad exposure of the wound area will bring the infection quickly under control.

b. *Fingertip Abscess*
The excision of a small triangle of nail ensures drainage of the pus. The necrotic bed of the abscess is carefully curetted away (Figure 199a,b).

c. *Suppuration in the Nail Fold and below the Nail (Paronychia)*
Small, highly localized abscesses on the lateral nail fold, often following manicure injuries, quickly heal after the soft tissue is pushed back from the nail. All necrotic tissue must be curetted away. If the entire nail fold is affected, longitudinal incisions are made bilaterally such that damage to the matrix is avoided. The nail fold is lifted, and necrotic tissue is removed. If the matrix is already involved in the purulent process,

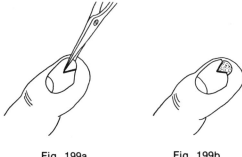

Fig. 199a   Fig. 199b

the nail must be removed. A layer of ointment gauze is loosely inserted beneath the lifted nail fold, covering the nail bed (Figure 200a–c).

d. Pustule in the Skin of the Finger
(Cutaneous Panaritium)

The pustule is completely removed with a scissors. The exposed corium is then closely inspected to see whether the surface pustule is connected by a small passage with a deeper subcutaneous abscess (collarbutton abscess; Figure 201).

A misdiagnosis can have devastating consequences for the finger. The process may spread to infect the bone and terminal joint, with subsequent involvement of the flexor tendon sheaths and joints at the middle and basal joints, and interdigital phlegmons at the proximal phalanx through involvement of the web skin creases and lumbrical canals. The mere suspicion of the presence of deep purulence is sufficient grounds for extending the operation.

e. Pulp Abscess (Subcutaneous Panaritium
of the Distal Phalanx)

The bulb of the finger is opened by a half frogmouth incision made close to the nail (Figures 198–1, 202). The orthodox curved incision far

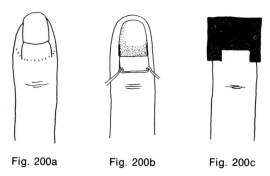

Fig. 200a   Fig. 200b   Fig. 200c

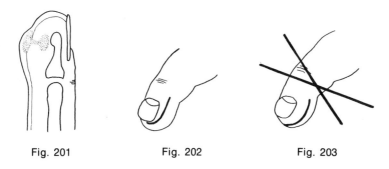

Fig. 201   Fig. 202   Fig. 203

from the nail leads to disturbances of sensation and blood flow and leaves behind troublesome scars (Figure 203). The incision should lie on the ulnar side of the second, third, and fourth fingers, and on the radial side of the thumb and little finger. All necrotic tissue is carefully removed. The wound is kept open if necessary with an oleaginous ointment gauze. Sometimes the abscess threatens to perforate the skin of the finger, or the pus has already been discharged. It is better in such cases to enter at the site of the perforation, with the incision following the skin cleavage lines. If a troublesome scar results, it can be corrected later. If the bulb of the finger is also opened from the side in such cases, the skin bridge may become necrotic.

f. Subcutaneous Suppuration of the Middle and Proximal Phalanges (Subcutaneous Digital Panaritium)

If the process is limited strictly to *one* phalanx, it is opened by a longitudinal volar incision (Figure 198–2). Crossing of a flexion crease leads to contracture and must thus be avoided. A sparing oval excision of the skin margin is permitted. In this way the wound will remain open and necrotomy will be facilitated. If both phalanges are involved, the incision lies mediolateral and dorsal to the neurovascular bundles, which must by all means be spared (Figure 198–3). Beware of opening the uninvolved flexor tendon sheath. Opening the volar side of the finger by the V- or W-shaped incision of Bruner provides excellent access but is dispensable in septic hand surgery.

g. Tendon Sheath Phlegmons (Panaritium Tendovaginosum)

Prompt diagnosis is essential for the preservation of finger function. Destruction of the sensitive gliding tissues in the tendon sheath through ischemic necrosis resulting from increased pressure leads to flexor tendon adhesions and promotes the spread of the infection to the tendon itself. The end result of this is tendon necrosis. A well-founded suspicion based on the flexed position of the fingers and pressure sensitivity in the course of the tendon sheath justifies operative intervention. It should be realized that tendon sheath phlegmons of the second and fourth fingers may invade the palmar space. In cases of phlegmons of the first and fifth fingers, V-phlegmons may occur, or the process may spread to the radial or ulnar tendon sheath sac proximal to the wrist and to the deep fascial space of the forearm on the interosseous membrane (Parona's space) (Figure 204).

The following situations occur:

i. Primary infection of the tendon sheath (*direct injury*): Through drainage is the therapy of choice. The tendon sheath must be opened in the flexion crease of the terminal joint by a transverse incision (Figure 198–4) and at the proximal end of the tendon sheath sac. For fingers two through four, the sheath is thus opened in the distal palmar flexion crease, also by transverse incision (Figure 198–5), and for fingers one and five at the forearm proximal to the wrist by a longitudinal incision over the ulna dorsal to the ulnar flexor muscle of the wrist (Figure 198–6). A venoflex catheter is inserted into the tendon sheath up to the level of the middle joint if possible. The distal end of the tendon sheath is also held open by a short plastic catheter (Figure 205). Irrigation of the tendon sheath with a single instillation of 1 million units of penicillin G is generally sufficient. If this is insufficient to control the infection, the sheath is irrigated again after 6 hours with 0.5–1.0 ml of a 0.5% solution of neomycin until the fluid discharge is clear. Two days later the drains are removed. This type of purulence has a poor prognosis in terms of function.

ii. Secondary infection of the tendon sheath: This is usually accompanied by extensive suppuration of the finger pulp, which must be removed at operation. This is best done by making a mediolateral incision on the finger and opening the tendon sheath, taking care to spare the annular ligaments. At the same time, a through drain is introduced as described. On

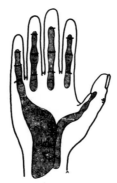

Fig. 204

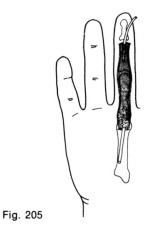

Fig. 205

the thumb and little finger, it may be necessary to extend the incisions along the eminence to the forearm. In the process, the carpal canal is split in order to relieve pressure on the flexor tendons and median nerve (Figure 198–7).

After the operation the fingers are immobilized in flexion by means of a dorsal plaster splint until the infection is safely under control. If tendon necrosis has occurred, as evidenced by a gray-green discoloration of the tendon tissue, the infection cannot be halted until the last tendon sequestrum is removed. The scar formation following prolonged suppuration dooms reconstructive tendon surgery to failure from the start, however. Necrotic tendons must therefore be promptly removed.

h. Suppuration in the Fascial Spaces
   of the Hand and Forearm
   There are six spaces in which suppuration may occur:

1) The deep palmar space, bounded volarward by the flexor tendons, radialward by the third metacarpal, and ulnarward by the hypothenar.
2) The thenar space in the region of the thenar musculature.
3) The hypothenar space in the region of the hypothenar musculature.
4) The dorsal subcutaneous space dorsal to the extensor tendons.
5) The dorsal subaponeurotic space between the extensor tendons and the metacarpals.
6) Parona's space in the forearm, situated between the long flexors, the quadrate pronator muscle, and the interosseous membrane.

i. Note on Space 1: The deep palmar space is opened by a curved cutaneous incision with section of the palmar aponeurosis (Figure 198–8).

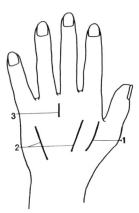

Fig. 206

ii. Note on Space 2: The thenar space is accessible on the volar side by incision parallel to the thenar crease (Figure 198–7), and on the dorsal side by a curved incision on the radial border of the first dorsal interosseous muscle (Figure 206–1). *Beware of injury to the motor branch of the median nerve at the thenar!* The first interdigital crease must not be sectioned lest adductive contraction occur.

iii. Note on Space 3: The hypothenar space (rarely affected) is approached from a longitudinal volar incision, splitting the fascia (Figure 198–9).

iv. Note on Spaces 4 and 5: The two fascial spaces on the dorsum of the hand are opened by two longitudinal incisions at the radial and ulnar border of the extensor bundle (Figure 206–2).

v. Note on Space 6: Parona's space is exposed on the radial side by a longitudinal incision between the brachioradial muscle and the radius, and on the ulnar side between the ulnar flexor muscle of the wrist and the ulna (Figure 198–10). The entire forearm fascia must be split in order to decompress the median nerve.

In the treatment of fascial space suppuration, draining the pus does not free the surgeon from the obligation of removing all necrotic tissues (while sparing important anatomical substrates). Postoperative treatment with through drainage has proved to be an effective supportive measure. If the cutaneous incisions are extensive, the delayed primary suture can generally be safely employed under the protection of through drainage and general antibiotic therapy.

i. Callus Abscess and Interdigital Phlegmons
These infections are often accompanied by an extensive, somewhat reddened edema of the dorsum of the hand. This should not prompt a

primary dorsal incision just because the palm appears unremarkable at first sight. The callosity in this region conceals all the signs of inflammation except pain. A careful search for the pus cavity with a bulb-headed probe (circumscribed pain) will guard against errors. Of course, collar-button-like perforations to the dorsal side are as likely to occur as invasions of the deep palmar space.

The interdigital creases must be spared when the abscess is opened. The incision is curved, following the hand lines in the region of the affected callus (Figure 198–11). Palmar aponeurotic tissue is resected, and necrotic tissues are carefully removed. The wound is kept open by a sparing oval excision of skin. A dorsal counterincision is rarely needed, but when needed it is made in the form of a longitudinal cut central to the interdigital crease. A rubber strip is pulled through for drainage (Figure 206–3).

j. Pyarthrosis (Suppuration in the Joints)

Diagnosis is based on swelling and intense pain on motion. In the early stage, an attempt is made to treat the condition by daily punction on the dorsal side and the instillation of an antibiotic while the member is fixed by plaster in the position of function. If x-ray changes are evident, especially a narrowing of the joint space as an expression of cartilage destruction or bony defects, operative intervention is warranted. The terminal and middle joints are best opened by mediolateral incision, but may be opened from the dorsal side, requiring that the extensor tendons be drawn back from the operating area. The articular surfaces are resected completely but as sparingly as possible; the capsule is also excised. Then stiffening will either occur spontaneously or must be produced operatively at the terminal and middle joints. At the basal joint, resection of the head of the associated metacarpal often yields remarkably good functional results. Empyema of the wrist requires broad exposure of the joint, preferably from the ulnar side with section of the ulnar extensor and flexor muscles of the wrist. Aftercare supported by through drainage will shorten the treatment time. In the case of an advanced infection of the finger joint subsequent to panaritium tendovaginosum, amputation is generally unavoidable unless the affected digit is the thumb.

k. Suppuration of the Bone (Panarithium Ossale, Fracture Osteitis)

This condition is usually associated with an advanced infection or osteitis following an open fracture. Hematogenic osteomyelitis plays only a minor role in the hand. In the advanced bone infection, the clinical picture is dominated initially by the symptoms of pulp and tendon sheath infection. Only later do persistent fistulas give clear evidence of bone infection. Fistular suppuration as well as delayed union are characteristic of fracture osteitis. As in any bone infection, an early diagnosis cannot be made on the basis of x-ray evidence. In panaritium ossale, clear x-ray signs do not appear before 1 week, and in fracture osteitis, 2 weeks. Osteolysis with the formation of partial or total sequestra is the predominant feature. The necrotic bone becomes rich in calcium shortly before detachment, in contrast to adjacent bone, which is still well perfused and thus lower in calcium. In the case of total sequestration, the neighboring joints are usually involved as well.

Popkirow is correct when he says that bone purulence following the operative treatment of panaritia of the soft tissues can spoil a flawless operating technique. The best treatment is therefore prophylaxis.

i. Treatment in the x-ray–negative phase: The operative procedure is restricted to the soft tissues. Pus is drained and necrotic tissue is carefully removed. Immobilization is mandatory. The treatment is supported with antibiotics, without reliance on them.

ii. Treatment in the x-ray–positive phase: Sequestrotomy is employed with careful evidement of the granulation bed. In total sequestration, the complete or partial amputation of the finger is indicated. Only the thumb should be treated conservatively. In other words, the pulp of the thumb must be preserved, with bone or without. The amputation of the proximal phalanx of the index finger should also be avoided if possible. Sequestered carpal bones are removed.

l. Furuncles and Carbuncles

Lancing alone is insufficient, because the suppuration that persists in the presence of necrotic tissue endangers the function of the hand. A furuncle or carbuncle therefore must be excised. The resultant granulation surface is promptly covered with a Reverdin graft.

II. Primary Phlegmonous Infection

Highly virulent and invasive pathogens lead to a rapidly ascending lymphangitis and lymphadenitis, and in some cases to generalized septic phenomena. The most important of these pathogens are the streptococci, the mixed groups that occur in human and animal bite wounds, and perianal coliforms.

Two disease forms are especially common in daily practice: erysipelas and erysipeloid. Both diseases produce a sharply circumscribed redness, that of erysipelas often appearing darker and sometimes almost bluish red. Erysipelas, however, begins with generalized septic phenomena (chills, high fever), while erysipeloid rarely becomes generalized and occurs almost exclusively in persons having occupational contact with meat or fish.

Primary phlegmonous infections are less common than pyogenic infections, but the physician must be familiar with them so that he can draw correct therapeutic conclusions from his diagnosis. Unlike the pyogenic infection, the primary phlegmonous infection should be treated chiefly with high doses of antibiotics, with surgical measures assuming a secondary role in the event of liquefaction or in the primary care of bite wounds. This surgery, incidentally, is governed by the same rules that apply to the pyogenic infection.

The following antibiotics are preferred in the treatment of primary phlegmonous infections:

Penicillin G (up to 60 million units/24 hours), combined with gentamycin if desired.
Synthetic penicillins.
Tetracyclines.
Erythromycin.

Bite wounds merit particular attention in this regard, inasmuch as there is a likelihood of infection with anaerobic microorganisms. Wound excision should therefore be followed by delayed primary suture to guard against unpleasant surprises. In many areas the possibility of rabies must also be considered. The best prophylactic measure is the prompt, thorough washing of the wound with hexachlorophene. Do not disinfect the wound with alcohol disinfectants! Cleansing is followed by careful excision of the wound. The necessity of administering rabies vaccine must be decided on a case-by-case basis.

III. Differential Diagnosis

The surgeon must not confuse the painless primary lesion of syphilis with pyogenic paronychia, and should also consider the possibility of mycosis, which requires appropriate aftercare. Other diseases that must be considered during differential diagnosis are: vascular diseases (Raynaud's disease), diabetes mellitus, trophic disturbances following peripheral nerve lesions, diseases of the central nervous system, syringomyelia, sarcoidosis, and glomic tumors. Tuberculosis is yet another possibility. Its x-ray evidence may cause it to be confused with hematogenic osteomyelitis. Since it tends to appear primarily in the region of the hand and only rarely presents the organic manifestation of a generalized tuberculous infection, its recognition is also important in terms of patient insurance.

IV. Reconstructive Surgery following Hand Infections

The extent of the functional disabilities following infections of the hand depends to a large degree on the time at which treatment is begun. Even the best treatment cannot always prevent motor impairments due to scar contractures, tendon damage, ankylosis, bone deformities and defects, pseudarthrosis, sensory disturbances and losses, or amputations. To minimize these losses of function, measures must be taken that range from the restoration of a stress-resistant integument to major operations with the object of constructing substitute forms of grasp. There are no standard procedures for improving the sequelae to hand infections. Instead, the operations follow the basic rules of reconstructive surgery with regard for general surgical principles. They must be planned with great care. The beginner should exercise extreme restraint in this area, but he should know the possibilities for reconstruction so that he can properly guide and advise his patient.

A. Skin

Granulating wound surfaces jeopardize the success of any operation on deep anatomical substrates (tendons, nerves, bones) due to the increased danger of infection. Extensive granulations are therefore covered with split-skin grafts and small ones with Reverdin grafts.

Poorly perfused scar tissue is also replaced with split-skin or full-thickness grafts. If tendon or bone repair is planned in such areas, a pedicle flap is preferred.

Contracted scars are corrected by flap advancement (Z-plasty, etc.).

B. Bones

Malunions require osteotomy. Pseudarthrosis and defects are corrected with autologous bone grafts, preferably from the iliac crest. For osteosynthesis, Kirschner wires are best.

C. Joints

If a joint is ankylosed in a faulty position and is painful or unstable, arthrodesis in the position of function is the procedure of choice. Even the arthrodesis of both interphalangeal joints in a favorable position only slightly diminishes the functional value of the finger. If the middle and basal joints are affected, arthrodesis of the middle joint combined with arthroplasty of the basal joint or resection of the metacarpal head can produce satisfactory results. We consider alloarthroplasty problematic on general principles, especially following an infection, and can envision no case in which it would be warranted in the hand.

D. Tendons

The transfer of flexor tendons remains problematic despite the progress made in this field, and it is especially difficult following an infection of the sheath with tendon necrosis. On the whole, our results with this procedure have been disappointing. Because the result achieved by flexor tendon transfer can be obtained better and more rapidly by arthrodesis, such a transfer is indicated only under exceptionally favorable circumstances. The situation is similar to that involving the extensor apparatus of the fingers, although the replacement of the common extensor has good prospects for success.

E. Nerves

A sensory transfer is indicated more often than secondary nerve suture or a nerve graft. The most common syndrome is the symptomatic nerve compression syndrome (usually of the median nerve, occasionally of the ulnar nerve) following an infection of the fascial spaces. This syndrome is treated by decompression of the nerve in the carpal canal or canal of Guyon.

F. Creation of Secondary Forms of Grasp following Finger Losses

The possibilities are discussed in the chapter on Amputations. An additional point should be mentioned, however. A finger that is due for amputation because of flexor tendon necrosis, empyema of the middle joint, and sequestering osteitis of the proximal phalanx but still has sensation and a blood supply can be successfully pollicized by Hilgenfeldt's method despite florid infection, the destroyed structures being sacrificed in the process. A personal, previously unpublished case has demonstrated the success of this operation.

Bibliography

Adams, R. M., et al.: Hautinfektion mit Mycobacterium marium durch tropische Fischaquarien (Ref.). JAMA 211, 457 (1970).

Bolton, H., Fowler, P. J., Jepson, R. P.: The natural history and treatment of pulp space infections and osteomyelitis of the terminal phalanx. J. Bone Joint Surg. B 31, 499 (1949).

Büchter, L., Mörl, M.: Die eitrigen Entzündungen der Hand. Aetiologie, Verlaufsformen and funktionelle Spätergebnisse. Zentralbl. Chir. 89, 1711 (1964).

Entin, M. A.: Infections of the hand. Surg. Clin. North Am. 44, 981 (1964).

Heckstock, H.: Die eitrigen Sehnenscheidenentzündungen der Hand. Behandlung, Ergebnisse. Akt. Chir. 2, 285 (1967).

Hentschel, M.: Moderne Aspekte der septischen Handchirurgie. Chirurg 40, 403 (1969).

Huber, O., Tipold, E.: Behandlung der eitrigen Sehnenscheidenentzündung durch Spüldrainage. Akt. Chir. 5, 161 (1970).

Kanaval, A. B.: Study of acute phlegmons of the hand. Surg. Gynecol. Obstet. 1, 221 (1905).

Koob, E.: Wiederherstellungsoperationen an der Hand nach Infektionen. Hefte Unfallheilkd. 107, 230 (1971).

Kress, H.: Bedeutung der aufgeschobenen Primärversorgung für die Behandlung infizierter Handverletzungen. Hefte Unfallheilkd. 107, 245 (1971).

Kühn, H. G.: Infektiöse Komplikationen bei Handverletzungen. Chir. Plast. Reconstr. 6, 54 (1969).

Popkirow, St.: Zur Diagnose und Therapie von Knocheninfektionen der Hand. Hefte Unfallheilkd. 107, 225 (1971).

Porras, C., et al.: Recovery from rabies in man. Ann. Intern. Med. 85, 44 (1976).

Rahmel, R.: Desolate Ergebnisse infolge infizierter Bagatellverletzungen an der Hand. Hefte Unfallheilkd. 107, 251 (1971).

Scott, J. C., Jones, B. V.: Results of treatment of infections of the hand. J. Bone Joint Surg. B 34, 581 (1952).

Stone, N. H., et al.: Empirical selection of antibiotics for hand infections. J. Bone Joint Surg. A 51, 899 (1969).

Titze, A.: Die akute eirige Sehnenscheidenentzündung. Chir. Praxis 11, 587 (1967).

Verth, M. zur: Das Panaritium. Ergeb. Chir. Orthop. 16, 653 (1923).

Willenegger, H., Roth, W.: Die antibakterielle Spüldrainage als Behandlungsprinzip bei der chirurgischen Infektion. Dtsch. Med. Wochenschr. 87, 1485 (1962).

Wilson, M. et al.: Presenting features and diagnosis of rabies. Lancet, 1139 (1975).

Thermal, Chemical, and Electrical Injuries

In these injuries the procedure is determined by the patient's general condition and the areal extent of the injury. The preservation of life must be our paramount concern in all extensive burns, but we need not abandon our concerns for the recovery of important motor functions. This is especially true for the hand, which is involved in a high percentage of all burn cases.

We shall deal here only with the management of local thermal or chemical injuries of the hand, rather than the "burn sickness," or generalized reaction to burn injuries. Even in isolated burns of the hand, however, the basic features of the general therapy of the burn sickness must by no means be neglected.

The primary general measures are as follows (as needed):

1) Treatment for initial shock (low molecular weight dextrans).
2) Pain relief (intravenous only, because the absorption conditions cannot be estimated for analgesics administered subcutaneously).
3) Fluid balance.
4) Tetanus prophylaxis.

From a surgical standpoint, the cause of the skin destruction, be it thermal or chemical, is of secondary importance since (with certain exceptions) all such injuries are characterized by coagulation necrosis. We shall therefore refer to these injuries as "burns," pointing out exceptions as they arise (e.g., colliquative necrosis brought on by certain chemicals, ischemic reaction to electric current and cold).

I. Diagnosis

The correct assessment of the extent of the burn is of eminent importance: the physician must know whether the epithelial elements of the skin have been completely destroyed or are partially intact. Remaining appendages of the skin and deep epithelial papillae permit a spontaneous, multicentric epithelialization which guarantees a sufficiently stress-resistant integument after healing. If all epithelial structures are destroyed, only a secondary epithelium can form by granulation from the edges of the wound, *but secondary epithelium is always inferior*. It may be acceptable in certain areas of the body that are subjected to little or no functional stresses, but *not in the hand*, due to the constant danger of cicatricial keloid formation. The contractural tendency of healing granulation tissue also jeopardizes the function of the hand.

It is therefore useful to classify burn cases according to two degrees of severity (Jackson, 1953):

1) Partial skin necrosis.
2) Total skin necrosis.

Partial skin necrosis is anemable to conservative therapy and should be treated accordingly.

Total skin necrosis should be considered a surgical wound that is largely free from infection when fresh and is therefore amenable to primary closure.

We can thus draw the following important therapeutic conclusions for the burned hand:

1) The primary treatment of partial skin necrosis is conservative. Necrotic skin areas may later require grafting to correct functionally disabling cicatrization, especially in children.
2) Total skin necrosis requires plastic repair as soon as possible in the interests of function.

However, even the very experienced hand surgeon may find it difficult to determine accurately the areal extent and especially the depth of burns immediately after the accident. The accident anamnesis, however, can be a valuable aid in interpreting the clinical evidence:

1) Very brief exposure to heat or hot liquids generally causes a partial necrosis of the skin. The clinical signs are redness and vesication. The loss of epidermis leaves a strongly secreting, well-perfused wound surface with intact pain receptors.

2)   Contact with hot objects, molten metals, and flames typically leads to total skin necrosis. Clinically, the burn shows the grayish white discoloration indicative of deep coagulation necrosis. The vessels are filled with stagnant blood. The affected areas are nonpainful due to the destruction of sensory nerve endings. The tissue has a leathery texture.

3)   Caustic liquids tend to produce total skin necrosis, especially if hot.

4)   In electrical injuries the degree of tissue damage depends on the strength of the current. Tendons and bones may be necrotized in such injuries.

5)   Certain chemical compunds lead to a progressive colliquative necrosis (e.g., hydrofluoric acid) or to severe generalized reactions combined with skin damage, even if the area of tissue contact is small (e.g., ethylenimine).

6)   Exposure to cold leads to local ischemia and thus to partial or total tissue necrosis.

Finally, vital coloration can be used as an index for determining the areal extent and the depth of total skin necrosis. Tempest's method using disulphine blue has proved practicable and adequate in this regard. The dye is supplied ready to inject in 10-ml ampules (Table 2). With slow intravenous injection, well-perfused skin areas such as the lips, face, and ears turn a deep blue-green in 60–90 seconds, and the entire body in 3–5 minutes. Devitalized tissue shows no color change. The dye is excreted with the urine in 3–4 days, depending on fluid intake and renal function. The patient must be informed of the anticipated color changes before the dye is injected.

The results of the test must be determined immediately after the dye has spread throughout the skin—and thus intraoperatively—before it has diffused into the burn edema. The test can be employed only if the circulatory conditions are intact. Impending or manifest shock is an absolute contraindication. The vital coloration test is useful only if one is willing and able to draw immediate therapeutic (i.e., operative) conclusions from the result. The operation must therefore already be prepared.

TABLE 2.   Dosage of Disulphine Blue[a]

Age (yr)	Dose (ml)
3 or younger	5–10
3–10	10–15
10–20	20
Over 20	20–40

[a] Manufacturer: Imperial Chemical Industries Ltd.

II. Therapy

A. General Measures

The principal goal of the local treatment of burn wounds is the preservation of hand function. The sooner the wound is closed, whether by spontaneous epithelialization in partial skin necrosis or by grafting in total skin necrosis, the better the chance of successful preservation.

The burn wound is threatened by many dangers that interfere with rapid healing and the preservation of function:

1) Infection.
2) Edema.
3) Secondary thrombosis of small vessels.
4) Iatrogenic injuries.

Infection, edema, and thrombosis may develop into a vicious cycle and, especially when combined with improper measures, may transform a partial necrosis into a total necrosis, which may then spread to deeper structures, particularly on the dorsal side of the fingers.

1. Infection

The best treatment for infection is the prophylaxis of bacterial contamination of the initially germ-free burn wound, especially with resistant hospital strains.

1) Primary general measures (see above), examination, and treatment must be carried out in an aseptic operating room with sterile clothing, surgical masks, and sterile rubber gloves. These precautions should also be observed in the office of the general practitioner to the fullest extent possible in the case of small superficial burns.

2) The bacterial contamination of granulating wound surfaces is unavoidable in the long run. They must therefore be promptly covered with skin. Inadequate precautions against infection jeopardize the success of plastic surgery, especially when free grafts are used.

3) Parenterally or enterally administered antibiotics are poorly suited in the long run for infection prophylaxis in burn cases. They are better suited for infectious complications that arise during the course of treatment. Regular bacteriological inspections of larger wounds are necessary in order to monitor the rapid bacterial changes that occur.

4) Local chemotherapeutic or antibiotic measures for the prophylaxis or treatment of infection are useful if they are instituted promptly

(i.e., at the start of treatment), and if they are limited to pathogens with low resistance. Sulfamylon, gentamycin, and neomycin in ointment form are recommended.

2. Edema

The local treatment occasionally recommended for the unavoidable edema phase in compression bandage therapy is not without its dangers even if correctly administered under clinical observation. Decompression of the edema by longitudinal incisions on the dorsum of the hand is preferred. It avoids further tissue damage resulting from strangulation of the vessels.

3. Secondary Thrombosis

In addition to disturbances of the microcirculation, edema and infection are the main causes of secondary thrombosis in the small vessels. Awareness of this fact can prevent the progression of skin necrosis.

4. Iatrogenic Injuries

a. During Initial Treatment

i. Disregard for infection prophylaxis

ii. Coarse brushing of the wound surface: This procedure was formerly recommended. This leads to the destruction of surviving islands of tissue.

b. During the Course of Treatment

i. Conservative treatment: A choice must be made between open or closed treatment of the wound. Open treatment is advantageous mainly in deep burns prior to the demarcation of necrotic tissue, provided daily supervised physical therapy can be promptly initiated. A disadvantage is the increased risk of infection. Edema, however, may force the basal finger joints into extension, thereby causing a shortening of the lateral ligaments which will endanger the later function of the hand. Hence, closed treatment is preferred for wounds of the hand, with the hand bandaged to maintain the position of function. The wrist is fixed in 30° dorsiflexion by a plaster splint. A ball of synthetic cotton or steel wool is placed in the palm. Gauze compresses protect the lateral surfaces of the fingers and prevent cicatricial syndactyly. The hand is elevated to promote mobilization of the edema. In exceptional cases, and especially in the open treatment of the hand in severe general burns, temporary drill-wire arthrodesis may be warranted (especially arthrodesis of the metacarpophalangeal joints in the position of function). It should be employed during the initial treatment if possible, in order to avoid deep bacterial contamination. Closed treatment in an ointment bandage requires daily (aseptic) bandage changes and cleansing to prevent tissue damage by maceration.

ii. Debridement: Too much conservatism in the treatment of total skin necrosis leads to unavoidable infection which will spread to deeper tissues. On the dorsal side of the hand, this means necrosis of the tendons and joint capsules. The volar side is in less danger from all but contact burns due to the resistance of the palmar fascia. Prompt necrotomy prevents excessive granulations and thus secondary contractures.

This leads to the following therapeutic conditions: If, for diagnostic or general medical reasons, one cannot decide on immediate operative treatment, necrotoym is carried out on the dorsal side followed at once by plastic repair on the third or fourth day after the accident. The surgery is performed in a bloodless field (tourniquet ischemia). The edema facilitates the removal of burned tissue from the intact substrate. The blood vessels provide a further guide for recognizing the boundaries of total necrosis: they are filled with blood in the burned tissue, but are empty in intact tissue due to the presence of the tourniquet. Spontaneous demarcation will occur on the volar side due to the thicker skin cover and the palmar fascial barrier. Devitalized tissue is removed at once. Only in deep contact burns is surgical intervention on the third or fourth day advised due to the danger of tendon, nerve, and vascular damage.

B. Treatment of Partial Skin Necrosis

1. Initial Treatment

a. Removal of Contaminants

Atraumatic removal of contaminants is performed with sterile physiological saline. Hot tar contaminants are better left alone, as the layer of tar will fall away by itself in a few days.

b. Removal of Epidermal Remnants

Epidermal remnants are removed immediately with scissors and tweezers. Blisters are removed down to their edges.

Measures a and b are carried out under anesthesia if necessary.

c. Bandaging

The wounds are covered with nonadherent gauze, then the hand is bandaged in the position of function for 8 to 10 days if no infection occurs (i.e., if the bandage remains dry).

d. Infection Prophylaxis

If prompt local infection prophylaxis is chosen, the local treatment is also carried out in a fist bandage, which must then be changed daily. The medication and wound secretions are washed off in luke-warm physiological saline.

e. Soothing Gels

In the case of superficial, or first-degree, burns, the application of antihistamine-containing gels has a very soothing effect. After the medication has dried, these burns can be treated further without bandaging or can be provided with a dry protective bandage.

Caution is advised in the treatment of children. Antihistamines are absorbed through the skin and may lead to intoxication in the sufficient doses.

f. Extensive Burns

The procedure just described is applied in the same way in extensive burns with involvement of the hand.

2. Further Treatment

a. Bandage Becomes Moist from the Inside

This may indicate infection. The bandage must be changed under sterile conditions. After the bandage is removed, the wound is first inspected. New blisters and tissue detritus are removed. It is determined whether the necrosis is progressing to deeper levels. After the first bandage is removed, daily bandage changes are needed until epithelialization has occurred.

b. Severe Edema Develops

Due to the danger of further tissue destruction, longitudinal incisions are made on the dorsum of the hand under anesthesia so that the edema can drain.

c. Wound Becomes Infected

Local antibiotic therapy is administered with daily bandage changes. Particular care should be taken to determine whether total necrosis has developed from partial necrosis, or whether the infection is progressing to deeper tissues and endangering important anatomical substrates.

General antiobiotic therapy is indicated, initially with high doses of penicillin (up to 60 million units/24 hours) until the pathogens and their resistances are determined. Beware of penicillin allergy.

Infection of the burn wound requires prompt necrotomy; it is advisable to combine surgical debridement with enzymatic debridement.

Beware of sepsis. It can have grave consequences, especially in children, even if the burn is quite small.

3. Aftercare

a. *Restoration of Hand and Finger Functions*

As a rule, the restoration of finger mobility presents no difficulties as long as the fingers are immobilized in the position of function. The threat of damage due to inactivity must be promptly recognized and corrected by physiotherapeutic measures. These may be instituted even before the wound has healed.

b. *Contractures and Keloids*

Scar contractures and keloids are to be expected even after partial skin necrosis with multicentric epithelial regeneration. They cannot be improved by physiotherapeutic and medicomechanical measures and may even be aggravated by them, inasmuch as the violent stretching of scar tissue leads to microhemorrhage into the tissue and thus to new fibroblastic activity. Contractures and keloids can be corrected only by plastic measures. In the case of keloids, which impair only the cosmetic outcome of surgery, a "wait and see" attitude is advised. In some cases a plastic correction is unnecessary when the atrophic scar stage is reached.

c. *Care of the Skin*

After the wounds have healed, and especially after washing, skin care by the generous application of oleaginous ointments (e.g., dexpanthenol ointment) or a simple oleaginour creme is indicated. This not only keeps tender new skin supple, but prevents detergent damage. When he resumes work, the patient should be urged to avoid exposure to coarse contaminants until the skin has regained its former toughness.

C. Treatment of Total Skin Necrosis

1. Hand Involvement in Extensive Burns of the Body

The procedure depends basically on the extent of the hand burn relative to the total extent of the burn injuries. If the hand must be treated within the context of extensive body burns, local measures are secondary to general treatment for burn sickness. We therefore limit ourselves to therapy as in partial skin necrosis. If circumstances permit, temporary drill-wire arthrodesis should be employed to maintain the position of function.

2. Isolated Burn of the Hand

In the case of an isolated hand burn, the damaged skin area may be regarded as an initially germ-free surgical wound that is amenable to immediate closure, provided the areas of total skin necrosis can be distinguished from healthy tissue on the basis of the clinical picture or vital coloration test. Primary surgery is not advised if it would endanger intact tissue as the result of uncertain demarcation. It is safer in such cases to administer immediate treatment according to the principles outlined above, and employ primary plastic measures on the third or fourth day according to the "emergency with delayed operation" principle, or even wait for spontaneous demarcation to take place.

a. Burn on the Dorsal Side

The dorsal burn is the simplest to evaluate in terms of areal extent and depth. At the same time, the deeper structures such as the tendons and finger joints are in much greater danger than on the volar side. The indications for primary plastic care, with which we have had the best results for some years, are quite broad. The excision may extend down to the gliding tissue of the extensor tendons, and the free grafts will still "take" with a high degree of certainty. Small contact burns are best repaired with Reverdin grafts, which are protected from the bandage with oleaginous ointment gauze. The hand is immobilized for 10 days in a foam rubber compression bandage. Larger areas are repaired with split-skin grafts. Care must be taken, especially in the case of the fingers, that the shrinking edges of the graft do not proceed in a longitudinal direction in such a way as to cause extension contractures. As desirable as open treatment may be with regard to the possibility of continuously monitoring the graft, only a few areas are amenable to fixation on a special splint (Larson). The grafts are therefore fixed with atraumatic sutures. The hand is then immobilized in a foam rubber compression bandage for 10 days. After the bandage is removed, secretions must be carefully daubed away daily until the graft is incorporated.

In the rare cases of tendon or bone involvement, pedicle flaps are essential. They must be adapted to the situation, and their transplantation follows the principles discussed in the chapter on the Care of Open Hand Injuries.

b. Burn on the Volar Side

For the reasons mentioned earlier, islands of epithelial tissue are often preserved that promote spontaneous regeneration. The palmar fascia acts as a protective barrier against the spread of the infection to deeper tissues. Since the palmar fascia must be removed before a graft can be applied, important anatomical structures are more endangered than protected by primary plastic measures. Closed treatment of the wound is therefore advised until demarcation has occurred, the latter being hastened by step-by-step surgical debridement. The wound is initally covered with split-skin grafts at the earliest possible time, but because these grafts are not always sufficiently stress resistant and are prone to shrinkage, especially in the palm area, secondary plastic measures are sometimes needed.

Only in deep contact burns exposing tendons, nerves, or bone is primary operative repair with pedicle flaps necessary.

c. Further Treatment

Free grafts are unbandaged after 10 days. In the case of pedicle flaps, the pedicle is sectioned after the third week. By the staged "training" of the flap (clamping the pedicle with a soft intestinal clamp or rubber tube starting at the end of the second week), the development of vascular attachments in the recipient bed is promoted.

An infection jeopardizes the success of the graft and may lead to flap necrosis. Necrotic grafts are removed and replaced by new grafts as soon as possible.

d. Aftercare

If skin closure is completed, an attempt must be made to restore hand funtion by intensive physiotherapeutic measures. If functional losses or deformities persist—usually due to scar contractures but possibly due to tissue defects on the dorsal side of the middle finger joints—surgical rehabilitation by prompt secondary operation is warranted.

e. Skin Care

This is as important for skin repaired by grafting as it is for burn wounds healed by spontaneous epithelialization.

D. Treatment of Special Types of Chemical Burn

As mentioned earlier, most chemical and thermal injuries result in coagulation necrosis of the skin, while a few substances lead to progressive colliquative necrosis despite an initial poverty of symptoms. The fate of the patient, however, does not depend on the chemical damage to the skin, but on the toxic effect of the compound on the body as a whole. Naturally, the physician and especially the surgeon cannot be expected to know the local action and general toxicity of all chemical compounds. *However, they are expected to obtain an accurate anamnesis (the patient is usually familiar with the properties of the substances with which he works), make a careful stationary observation of the patient in uncertain cases, and, if necessary, seek the assistance of an occupational hygienist, industrial physician, or detoxification center. The cause of many injuries can be determined by checking back with the patient's place of employment, even in the middle of the night!*

In view of the expansion of the chemical industry, every physician must deal with questions of toxicology at one time or another. It is beyond the scope of this book to discuss all the toxic compounds. Two prominent and fairly common examples will have to suffice:

1. Effects of Hydrofluoric Acid as an Example of Colliquative Necrosis

Hydrofluoric acid is widely used in the production of solvents, tanning agents, dyes, insecticides, and plastics, for surface treatment in the metal and glass industry, and in galvanizing. Workers in aluminum plants sometimes suffer "flux burns," which present a special disease picture known as the "electrolyte injury of furnace workers in the aluminum industry." The untreated hydrofluoric acid burn may lead to an extremely severe destruction of tissue, depending on the concentration. The process of tissue destruction and neutralization of the acid may continue for several days.

a. Symptoms

The main symptom is intense pain followed by erythema, edema, and colliquative necrosis within 1–24 hours, depending on the concentration. The necrosis may progress to deeper tissues within a period of several days and may invade the bone.

Thus, all the actions of chemical compounds on the skin require careful observation, even if the initial effect is pain accompanied by no apparent tissue lesion.

b. Therapy

Moeschlin, Thiele, and others recommend precipitation of the hydrofluoric acid in the tissue to insoluble calcium fluoride. Simon-Weidner disputes the efficacy of this therapy and advocates immediate surgical treatment. Based on personal experience, the latter treatment sometimes fails due to the difficulty of delineating the tissue damage clinically, whereas the "two-step therapy" of Thiele has proved effective if properly carried out. It is designed to precipitate hydrofluoric acid as insoluble calcium fluoride, prevent necrosis by calcium gluconate with hyaluronidase, and relieve pain with procaine.

Solution 1: A dry ampule of hyaluronidase is dissolved in 10 ml of 2% procain without adrenaline. The ready solution should contain at least 12 but not more than 17 I.U. hyaluronidase per milliliter.

Solution 2: In this solution 2% procaine and 20% calcium gluconate are mixed in equal parts, yielding a solution containing 1% procaine and 10% calcium gluconate.

Dose limits for procaine: The limits are 10 ml 2% and 20 ml 1% per injection; 30 ml 2% and 60 ml 1% per day. (For the treatment of toxic reactions, see the chapter on Anesthesia in Hand Surgery.)

The solutions are injected *successively* beneath the injured area with a thin cannula in a 1:2 ratio. Watch for ischemia due to fluid pressure, especially in the fingers. If mild pain recurs, reinjection with solution 2 is sufficient; otherwise both solutions are given. Treatment must be continued in this manner until the pain is gone. The necrosis that occasionally occurs, especially at high solution concentrations, is treated surgically. Affected fingernails must be removed immediately, since hydrofluoric acid permeates the nail.

In flux burns, two or three injections followed by prompt surgical treatment are generally sufficient to ensure problem-free healing.

Recent evidence suggests that the intra-arterial infusion of 10 ml of 20% calcium gluconate in 40 ml of 0.9% NaCl solution into the brachial artery over a 4-hour period improves the results of treatment.

> **The success of the treatment depends on its prompt commencement and correct continuance.**

---

2. Action of Ethylenimine as an Example of
   Chemical Skin Damage with Severe
   Generalized Toxic Reactions

This substance is not as widely used as hydrofluoric acid, but provides an instructive example. Despite 25 years of research and the analysis of two fatalities, the effects of percutaneous and inhalatory exposure on humans are not yet clearly known. It is known, however, that ethylenimine is highly toxic when taken in orally or through the skin, and extremely toxic when inhaled. The action of liquid ethylenimine on the skin can lead to total skin necrosis in a time period ranging from minutes to days, depending on the concentration. *This necrosis is treated according to surgical principles.*

Ethylenimine fumes have an irritating effect, particularly on the mucous membranes of the eyes and upper respiratory tract. They can also cause total necrosis in these areas.

Depending on the exposure time and concentration, inhalation of the substance can lead to periodic vomiting, glottic edema, pulmonary edema, and secondary bronchopneumonia.

The first attending physician must remember the following:

1) Especially when highly volatile substances are involved, percutaneous exposure may be accompanied by inhalation. The toxicological properties of the compound must be determined *immediately,* if necessary by making inquiry at the patient's place of employment.
2) Prompt referral to the internist, otorhinolaryngologist, and opthalmologist is indicated if the toxicology of a chemical substance suggests the possibility of actions beyond lesions of the skin.

E. Frostbite

Even the possibility of partial or total necrosis of the skin or deeper structures based on ischemia resulting from exposure to cold requires that the following general measures be taken simultaneously and *without delay:*

1) *Slow* warming of the entire body in cases of undercooling. *Caution:* The patient has lost his local thermoregulatory mechanisms and is therefore susceptible to local thermal injury.
2) Monitoring and regulation of the circulation. *Caution:* Opening the circulatory periphery may lead to a fall of blood pressure and shock.
3) Opening of the periphery and regulation of the microcirculation; intravenous infusion of low molecular weight dextrans with lencinocaine and Hydergine added.

The treatment of partial or total necrosis that has already developed is guided by the principles that generally apply to the treatment of thermal injuries.

F. Operative Reconstruction following Burns

1. Skin

Skin repair follows the general rules for producing a stress-resistant skin covering of the hand.

The following basic rules apply:

1) Scars that produce funiform contractures must be lengthened by single- or multistage Z-plasty. This gain in length is at the expense of width, however. The applications of this method are limited in the region of the fingers due to the danger of strangulation of the vessels.

2) On the dorsal side of the hand, two-thirds–thickness grafts (thick split-skin graft) can be used to create a stress-resistant integument as long as the defect to be repaired extends no deeper than the gliding tissues of the tendons. If sheath tissue is destroyed or if the bone is exposed, only a local pedicle flap or low-fat distant flap can be used.

3) On the volar side of the hand, a stress-resistant covering is best produced with pedicle flaps, although thick split-skin grafts and full-thickness grafts are also satisfactory. Distant pedicle flaps from the chest and abdomen must be used with caution, because if obesity develops later on, a fat pad will also form beneath the transplanted flap (depot fat). A better donor site is the contralateral inner surface of the upper arm, which has little depot fat.

4) Adductive contracture of the thumb due to a large scar in the first interdigital space requires repair by pedicle flap. A funiform scar can be lengthened by Z-plasty.

5) The other digital commisures are repaired by means of rotation flaps or split-skin grafts.

6) Insensible fingers that are immobile but still have a blood supply can be used to construct a skin covering after decortication of the bone.

7) Scar contractures at the edges of the graft must be avoided. It is desirable, therefore, that the edges of the graft (a) correspond to the course of the cleavage lines or creases of the hand, (b) are not rectilinear if possible and are not oriented in a longitudinal direction, and (c) follow the midlateral line of the fingers.

8) The hand must be in the position of function when free grafts are applied to the dorsal side.

9) Plastic repair of the palm is exceptional in that the hand is immobilized with the fingers extended and the thumb abducted. Aftercare of sufficient duration and continuity is especially important in this case.

10) The positions that must often be maintained during the healing of pedicle flaps sometimes lead to severe ankylosis. The physician should therefore be somewhat hesitant to use this form of dermoplasty on older patients and should determine whether a satisfactory result could be achieved more safely by the use of free grafts.

2. Proximal Interphalangeal Joints

The destruction of the intermediate tract leads to a flexion deformity of the proximal interphalangeal joints known as the "boutonnière deformity." Arthrodesis must generally be employed to restore a useful power grip.

3. Extension Stiffness of the Metacarpophalangeal Joints

This usually results from a shortening of the ligament apparatus, especially the lateral ligaments. An attempt can ba made to correct this condition, with varying degrees of success, by section or excision of the lateral ligaments of the metacarpophalangeal joints (see the chapter on Capsular Ligament Injuries).

4. Tendons

The plastic repair of tendon defects follows the rules of tendon surgery. A good skin covering and intact sheath must be present before plastic measures can be attempted, however. The technique should be applied with restraint.

5. Finger Losses

Secondary forms of grasp must be constructed by operative means, as described in the chapter on Amputations.

Bibliography

Dibbell, D. G., et al.: Hydrofluoric acid burns of the hand. J. Bone Joint Surg. A 52, 931 (1970).

Haynes, B. W.: Early excision and grafting in third degree burns. Ann. Surg. 736 (1969).

Larson, D. L., et al.: Repair of the boutonnière deformity of the burned hand. J. Trauma 10, 481 (1970).

Maisels, D. O.: The middle slip or boutonnière deformity in burned hand. Br. J. Plast. Surg. 18, 117 (1965).

Millesi, H.: Behandlungsergebnisse nach elektrischen Verbrennungen der Hände. Klin. Med. 22, 400 (1967).

Moeschlin, S.: Klinic und Therapie der Vergiftungen, 5. Aufl. Stuttgart: Thieme 1972.

Müller, F. E.: Hautplastiken in der Wiederherstellungschirurgie nach Verbrennungen. Chirurg 41, 398 (1970).

Schink, W.: Sofort- und Spätbehandlung thermischer Schäden der Hände. Münch. Med. Wochenschr. 105, 1452 (1963).

Seiffert, K. E.: Hautplastik bei der Versorgung frischer Verbrennungen. Chirurg 41, 393 (1970).

Simon-Weidner, R., Dreher, R.: Zur Behandlung der Flußsäureverätzungen. Med. Wochenschr. 19, 495 (1968).

Tempest, M. N.: Intravenöse Farbstoffinjektion zur klinischen Beurteilung der Lebensfähigkeit von Gewebe. Chir. Praxis 5, 265 (1961).

Thiele, W., Wild, H.: Die moderne Therapie der sog. „Flußverbrennungen". Praxis 51, 1097 (1962).

Thiess, A. M.: Gesundheitsschädigungen und Vergiftungen durch Einwirkung von Aethylenimin. Arch Toxikol. 21, 67 (1965).

Wittels, W.: Verbrennungsunfall beim Kind. Pädiat. Praxis 3, 290 (1967).

Hand Injuries in Children

In terms of operative technique, the same rules apply in the treatment of children as in the treatment of adults. However, the indications and tactics must be modified as the age of the patient decreases. They are influenced by the following factors:

I. Age

The younger the child, the more difficult the diagnosis.
The anamnesis must be obtained by a third party who is usually not even witness to the accident. An accurate examination is difficult if not impossible due to the child's reaction to the injury. Useful data on sensory losses cannot be obtained. If the child is asleep, some diagnostic evidence can be obtained on tendon injuries by comparing the position of injured fingers with adjacent fingers. Only the x-ray examination yields objective results if films are made of the healthy side for comparison. The diagnosis, however, depends ultimately on a correct and cautious operative procedure in which the surgeon must examine the nerves and tendons for continuity before the wound is closed. Only the experienced surgeon possesses the necessary skills for such an operation, particularly in view of the smallness of the structures involved.

II. Growth

Juvenile bone heals more rapidly and can compensate for malunions. The growth potential of juvenile tissue improves the prognosis of restorative operations on tendons and nerves. It thus favors the global restoration of all injured structures during primary care, especially since skin grafts tend to heal with fewer problems than in the adult. Tendons and nerves require urgent care to prevent atrophy of the fingers. Reoperations, especially on the tendons, have a better prognosis in the child.

Growth can have an adverse effect on scars, including of course scars at the edges of grafts. They cannot keep pace with the rapid growth of the hand and fingers during childhood and thus lead to contractures. This occurs regardless of the thickness of the graft. Thus, regular follow-up examinations are necessary for some years so that the need for corrective surgery can be promptly recognized.

III. Uncooperativeness

Small children normally lack the intelligence required for a structured program of therapeutic exercise. However, this lack is fully offset by the child's natural tendency to move about and play if uninhibited. The child can rehabilitate himself in this way (there is no "pension neurosis" or Sudeck's disease in children).

We thus see that the success of the treatment stands or falls with the operation. Operations on children therefore must be performed by experienced surgeons.

IV. Bandaging and Immobilization

The small anatomical relations and the restlessness of small children make the application of a secure bandage and immobilization difficult, especially in view of the fact that juvenile tissue is more susceptible than adult tissue to compressive injury. Our favorite technique is to place the child onto a T-shaped, well-padded wire splint arrangement on which the torso and abducted arms are fixed with wide elastic bands. The fingertips must remain visible so that the circulatory conditions can be monitored. Later a padded long arm case is used.

V. Summary

In summary, the following points must be considered in the treatment of hand injuries in children:

1) The success of treatment stands or falls with the operation.
2) The operations are for experienced surgeons only.
3) General anesthesia and tourniquet ischemia are essential.
4) The global restoration of all injured structures during primary care is desirable, thereby exploiting the favorable growth tendency of juvenile tissue.
5) The child's love of play must be exploited during physical therapy.
6) Years of follow-up examinations are needed to prevent loss of function due to scar contractures.

Bibliography

Millesi, H.: Wachstumsbedingte Narbenkontrakturen und ihre Bedeutung für die Handchirurgie. Langenbecks Arch. Chir. 299, 112 (1961).
Stelling, F. H.: Surgery of the hand in the child. J. Bone Joint Surg. A 45, 623 (1963).
Wakefield, A. R.: Hand injuries in children. J. Bone Joint Surg. A 46, 1226 (1964).

Sudeck's Disease

Dystrophy of the Extremities

The literature on this disease picture fills volumes. Even the definition is disputed. This is not the place to deal with theoretical problems, but the following features of the disease are of *practical* importance:

1) This neurogenic (and sometimes psychogenic), abacterial, inflammatory circulatory disorder may be a sequel to injury, depending on individual disposition.
2) The disease is potentiated by pain.
3) It affects *all* the tissues.
4) Remission is possible in stages I and II of the disease.
5) The disease may lead to the complete functional disability of the hand in stage III.

The course of the dystrophic process is characterized by three stages extending over a period of weeks or months:

I. Increased blood flow.
II. Diminished blood flow.
III. Diminished blood flow commensurate with the diminution of function.

Each stage can be correlated with a typical clinical picture:

I. Subjective: Feeling of heat, pain on motion.
    Objective: Swelling, redness, local temperature rise, hyperhidrosis, thickening of joint capsule with functional impairment of the joints, muscular atrophy, diffuse osteanabrosis.

II. Subjective: Feeling of cold.
     Objective: Cold pallor of the skin, leiodermia, persistence of functional losses, spotty decalcification of the bone.

III. Persistent functional losses due to joint stiffness with a delicate but otherwise harmonic or numerically diminished but intensified bony trabeculae pattern.

I. Diagnosis

Even the initial subjective and objective signs of abacterial inflammation during the course of treatment of a hand injury may indicate incipient dystrophy and must therefore be taken very seriously.

> **If the physician is not alerted to the condition until he finds atrophy of the bone, his diagnosis and thus his treatment are several weeks too late.**

II. Differential Diagnosis: Traumatic Edema of the Dorsum of the Hand

This condition occurs after trivial injuries and is characterized by a very firm swelling on the dorsum of the hand that may spread to the fingers. The x-ray shows no spotty demineralization. There is always the possibility that the swelling is the result of an artifact or self-inflicted injury. The therapy is immobilization in a circular plaster bandage. If the edema is associated with an autolesion, it will disappear. If it persists, a biopsy of the cutaneous and subcutaneous tissue must be performed to delineate the dermatologic disease picture.

III. Treatment

The best treatment is prevention by a well-structured program of active therapeutic exercise commencing on the day of the accident. If dystrophy is present, the course of action must be geared toward the progress of the disease.

A. Stage I

All measures are directed toward relieving pain and reducing the increased blood flow. Careful active exercise may be useful.

1) Immobilization with elevation of the extremity (position of function).
2) Medicinal treatment.
   a) Autonomic blockade.
   b) Antiphlogistics.
3) Hydrotherapy; the consensual reaction is exploited by cooling baths of the *healthy* arm.
4) Active therapeutic exercise safely *below* the threshold of pain; passive exercise or the local application of heat is not advised.

B. Stage II

The therapy is geared toward correcting the deficient blood flow and restoring articular function.

1) Medicinal treatment.
   a) Autonomic blockade.
   b) Vasodilating medication (Hydergine).
2) Hydrotherapy.
   a) Warming baths beginning with the healthy arm to exploit the consensual reaction.
   b) Warm (not hot) whirlpool baths.
3) Active therapeutic exercise below the pain threshold.

C. Stage III

By the classic definition, functional losses in this stage are irreversible. Nevertheless, efforts may be made to improve the condition by hydrotherapy, physical therapy, careful limbering of the joints, and active splinting.

> **The physician is warned against operative intervention! He, not the disease, will be blamed for failures.**

The transitions between stages I and II are not abrupt, and therapeutic measures should not be rigidly fixed according to the scheme above, but adapted to the situation. *Failure to recognize the situation can always provoke a relapse to stage I.*

IV. Prognosis

Prolonged impairments of function are not uncommon, and the treatment requires great patience from both doctor and patient. The prognosis must therefore be made with caution.

Bibliography

Blumensaat, C.: Der heutige Stand der Lehre vom Sudeck-Syndrom. Hefte Unfallheilkd. 51 (1956).
Sudeck, P.: Kollaterale Entzündungszustände (sog. akute Knochenatrophie und Dystrophie der Gliedmaßen) in der Unfallheilkunde. Hefte Unfallheilkd. 24 (1928).
Thorban, W.: Das Sudeck'sche Sydrom der Hand. Hefte Unfallheilkd. 75, 139 (1963).

Ischemic Contracture

A deficient blood supply due to external influences leads to the degeneration of muscle tissue with fibrosis and cicatricial contractures of the hand and fingers. Trauma plays a prominent causative role, whether by direct muscle damage due to electric shock or crush injury, edema of the muscle due to a loss of fascial and cutaneous stretch reserves, or a constricting bandage.

I. Diagnosis and Differential Diagnosis

A strict distinction must be made between Volkmann's contracture of the forearm, which should not be confused with combined median–ulnar palsy, and the more common ischemic contracture of the small hand muscles.

Volkmann's contracture leads to clawing with adduction of the thumb against the index finger, thereby creating a paralysis picture with the hand in the "intrinsic minus position." Increased flexion of the wrist opens the fingers (Figure 207).

For anatomical reasons, local ischemic contracture of the hand shows a completely different but nonetheless characteristic picture. Cicatricial contracture of the small hand muscles results in a slight flexion of the metacarpophalangeal joints of the long fingers ("intrinsic plus position") with extension of the middle and terminal joints, an increase in palmar convexity, and adduction of the thumb into the palm. This deformity interferes with closure of the fist and also prevents the hand from opening to grasp large objects (Figure 208).

The contracture may be limited to certain fingers or the thumb and

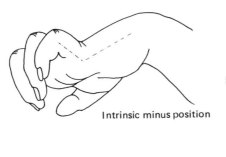

Fig. 207

Intrinsic minus position

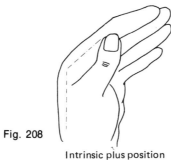

Fig. 208

Intrinsic plus position

can thus make diagnosis difficult. Clinically, it is distinguished from other forms of contracture by the fact that the three finger joints are freed from their inability to flex when the metacarpophalangeal joint is passively fixed in extension. At operation, the affected musculature shows a yellow-gray discoloration with characteristic cicatricial and fibrotic changes that are unmistakable. Incipient contracture is accompanied by unbearable ischemic pain which (fortunately) responds poorly to pain-relieving medication. Nevertheless, the onset of this complication is all too often unrecognized or overlooked, with the consequent failure to take immediate prophylactic or therapeutic measures.

II. Prophylaxis

Avoid constricting bandages.
Slit circular casts immediately to relieve pressure.
Elevate the extremity.
Treat for edema.
Institute therapeutic exercise program.

III. Treatment of Impending Contracture

Remove the cast or bandage.
Split the skin and fascia (lacertus fibrosus, forearm fascia, carpal canal, fascia of small hand muscles).

IV. Treatment of Fully Developed Contracture

A. Conservative Treatment

A program of therapeutic exercise is conducted under the direction of a physiotherapist and assisted by therapeutic splints. As a matter of principle, operative measures are preceded by conservative measures in both Volkmann's contracture and local contracture of the hand.

B. Operative Treatment

1. Volkmann's Contracture

Gosset's operation consists of deinsertion of all flexor musculature of the forearm.

2. Local Contracture of the Hand

Surgical treatment consists of deinsertion of the interossei from the metacarpal bones and tenotomy of the interosseous tendons (both susceptible to relapse). In addition, extirpation of the contracted interossei and excision of the oblique fibers of the lateral slips of the extensor aponeurosis (Littler) are performed (Figures 209, 210). All contracted muscles of the thumb must be removed. After the muscular contracture is eliminated, it is sometimes necessary to extend the skin covering of the first interdigital space by means of pedicle flaps.

C. Aftertreatment

Immobilization of the metacarpophalangeal joints in extension is instituted for 2 weeks, with immediate active movement of the interphalangeal joints. Intensive therapeutic is exercise guided by a physiotherapist

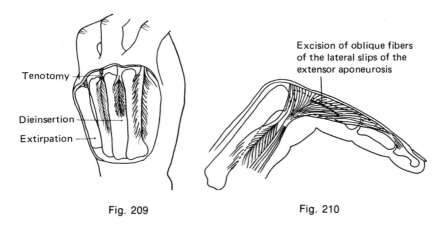

Tenotomy

Dieinsertion

Extirpation

Excision of oblique fibers
of the lateral slips of the
extensor aponeurosis

Fig. 209   Fig. 210

and supervised by the physician. Therapeutic and nocturnal splints are used.

V. Prognosis

Both forms of ischemic contracture, if fully developed, will result in some degree of functional disability in spite of reconstructive surgery.

Of paramount importance is the prevention of contracture, whose occurrence may also have legal consequences for the attending physician in view of the severe losses of function.

Bibliography

Düben, W.: Volkmannsche und lokale ischämische Kontraktur der Hand. Langenbecks Arch. Chir. 299, 109 (1961).

Harris, C., Riordan, D. C.: Intrinsic contracture in the hand and its surgical treatment. J. Bone Joint Surg. A 36, 10 (1954).

Jones, D. A.: Volkmann's ischemia. Surg. Clin. North Am. 50, 329 (1970).

Zancolli, E: Cirugia de la mano. Musculos intrinsecos. Prensa Med. Argent. 43, 1299 (1956).

Zancolli, E.: Tendon transfers after ischaemic contracture of the forearm. Am. J. Surg. 109, 356 (1956).

On the Informatory Obligation
of the Physician

The performance of an operation depends ultimately upon the consent of the patient. The procurement of this consent requires that the physician inform the patient of the typical risks, possible complications, and prospects for success. This is true for the care of a fresh injury as well as for plastic reconstructive measures.

The surgeon would do well to take his informatory obligation seriously, for failure to adequately inform the patient may have legal consequences.

We make it a practice in our clinic to ask each patient to sign a standard form confirming that he has been duly informed about the operation and has thereupon consented to it. Naturally this declaration of consent does not protect us from possible consequences if the operation fails or complications arise, but it does free the doctor from the considerable burden of proving that he has fulfilled his obligations if legal proceedings ensue.

Books and Monographs on Hand Surgery

Andina, F.: Die freien Hauttransplantationen. Berlin: Springer 1970.

Bailey, D. A.: The infected hand. London: Lewis 1963.

Biesalski, K., Mayer, L.: Die physiologische Sehnenverpflanzung. Berlin: Springer 1916.

Boyes, J. H.: Bunnell's surgery of the hand, 4th ed. Philadelphia: Lippincott 1964.

Buff, H. U.: Hautplastiken. Stuttgart: Thieme 1952.

Bunnell, St.: Surgery of the hand. Philadelphia: Lippincott 1944.

Bunnell, St.: Surgery of the hand, 5th ed. (Edited by J. H. Boyes). Philadelphia: Lippincott 1970.

Bürkle de la Camp, H., Schwaiger, M. (Hrsg.): Handbuch der gesamten Unfallheilkunde. Stuttgart: Ende 1963.

Converse, J. M. (ed.): Reconstructive plastic surgery. Philadelphia: Saunders 1964.

Crenshaw, A. H. (ed.): Campbell's operative orthopaedics. St. Louis: Mosby 1963.

Ender, J., Krotscheck, H., Simon-Weidner, R.: Die Chirurgie der Handverletzungen. Vienna: Springer 1956.

Eriksson, E.: Atlas der Lokalanaesthesie. Stuttgart: Thieme 1970.

Flynn, J. E. (ed.): Hand surgery. Baltimore: Williams and Wilkins 1966.

Gelbke, H.: Wiederherstellende und plastische Chirurgie. Stuttgart; Thieme 1963.

Häuptle, O.: Die aseptischen Chondro-Osteonekrosen. Berlin: de Gruyter 1954.

Heim, U., Pfeiffer, K. M.: Small fragment set manual: Technique recommended by the ASIF group. New York: Springer 1974.

Hilgenfeldt, O.: Operativer Daumenersatz und Beseitigung von Greifstörungen bei Fingerverlusten. Stuttgart: Enke 1950.

Iselin, M: Chirurgie de la main. Livre du chirurgien. Paris: Masson 1955.

Iselin, M.: Atlas de chirurgie de la main. Paris: Flammarion 1958.

Kanavel, A. B.: Infections of the hand, 7th ed. Philadelphia: Lea and Febiger 1940.

Kaplan, E. B.: Functional and surgical anatomy of the hand, 2nd ed. Philadelphia: Lippincott 1965.

Klapp, R., Beck, H.: Das Panaritium. Leipzig: Hirzel 1953.

Lange, M.: Die menschliche Hand. Stuttgart: Enke 1956.

Lanz, T. v., Wachsmuth, W.: Praktische Anatomie, Bd. I, 3. Berlin: Springer 1959.

Lexer, E.: Die freien Transplantationen. Stuttgart: Enke 1924.

McMinn, R. M. H., Hutchings, R. T.: A color atlas of human anatomy. London: Wolfe 1977.

Merle d'Aubigné, R., Benassy, J.: Chirurgie orthopédique des paralysies. Paris: Masson 1956.

Moberg, E.: Dringliche Handchirurgie. Stuttgart: Thieme 1964.

Moore, D. C.: Regional block. Springfield, Ill.: Thomas 1965.

Mumenthaler, M., Schliack, H.: Läsionen peripherer Nerven. Stuttgart: Thieme 1965.

Nigst, H.: Die Chirurgie der peripheren Nerven. Stuttgart: Thieme 1955.

Skoog, T.: The surgical treatment of burns. Stockholm: Almquist and Wiksell 1963.

Stockhusen, H., Hilgenfeldt, O.: Neue Erkenntnisse in der modernen Chirurgie der Hand. Stuttart: Enke 1970.

Sunderland, S.: Nerves and nerve injuries. Baltimore: Williams and Wilkins 1968.

Terminology for hand surgery. Brentwood: Westbury Press 1970.

Watson-Jones, R.: Fractures and joint injuries, 4th ed. Baltimore: Williams and Wilkins 1955.

Wilhelm, A.: Die Gelenkdenervation und ihre anatomischen Grundlagen. Hefte Unfallheilkd. 86 (1966).

Witt, A. N.: Sehnenverletzungen und Sehnenmuskeltransplantationen. Munich: Bergmann 1953.

Zenker, R., Heberer, G., Hegemann, G.: Allgemeine und spezielle chirurgische Operationslehre. Bd. X/3: Die Operationen an der Hand (hrsg. v. W. Wachsmuth u. A. Wilhelm). Berlin: Springer 1972.

Zrubecky, G.: Die Hand, das Tastorgan des Menschen. Stuttgart: Enke 1960.

Index